CW00822259

Once regarded diseases, diabetes today managed; it no longer restri productive life. Yet it cannot be treated with medication alone. The new methods of control require individual's close cooperation in developing a compatible and active lifestyle for a general reduction in high risk factors to supplement insulin therapy.

This excellent book provides all basic information about diabetes and diabetic control: its causes and types, importance of early detection, monitoring, high and low sugar emergencies, taking insulin through injection and tablets, the various Dos and Don'ts for skin, dental and eye care, and advise for pregnant women and diabetic children. Exhaustive meal planner with Calorie and Protein Exchange Charts is provided for scientific planning of nutritious and balanced diet.

'Provides fundamental explanations of the everyday problems of living with diabetes in a readable format.'

Melvin M Chertrack, MD, FACP
Past President, American Diabetes Association

The Author

Ada P. Kahn has a Master's degree in Public Health from Northwestern University Medical School, USA, and is a former member of the teaching faculty of the University of Health Sciences, Chicago Medical School and Columbia College, Chicago. She is a consultant to various pharmaceutical companies and medical associations. Her background includes affiliations with American Medical Association, the US Army Department of Medical History, and the US Department of Health and Human Services. She had worked with numerous health-related associations and organizations in educational capacities over the past 30 years.

She is a fellow of the American Medical Writers Association and the co-author of award winning Facts on File titles, *The Encyclopedia of Phobias, Fears and Anxieties, Midlife Health: A Woman's Practical Guide to Feeling Good,* and is the author of bestselling *Arthritis: Causes, Prevention and Treatment.*

Diabetes

Causes, Prevention and Treatment

Ada P Kahn
MPH

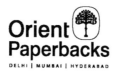

Orient
Paperbacks

DELHI | MUMBAI | HYDERABAD

Acknowledgements

The author thanks Melvin M. Chertack, MD, for his assistance
in making editorial changes to clarify some of the medical
explanations in this book. His cooperation has contributed
greatly to the readability of this book.

Thanks also to the Northern Illinois Affliate of the American
Diabetes Association for making current reference materials available
and to research assistant Ruth D. Kahn and Michael Kite.

www.orientpaperbacks.com

ISBN 13: 978-81-222-0034-7
ISBN 10: 81-222-0034-6

1st Published 1985
16th Printing 2007

Diabetes: Causes, Prevention & Treatment

© Ada P. Kahn, MPH 1983

Cover design by Vision Studio

Published by
Orient Paperbacks
(A division of Vision Books Pvt. Ltd.)
5A/8, Ansari Road, New Delhi-110 002

Printed in India at
Saurabh Printers Pvt. Ltd., Noida

Cover Printed at
Ravindra Printing Press, Delhi-110 006

Preface

We all have probably heard of Diabetes Mellitus or simply diabetes, without knowing precisely what this means. The word diabetes comes from the Greek language meaning 'to pass through, or to flow through', and mellitus means 'sweet'. Hence, it is merely a description of what is happening in the body: a fliud containing sugar passes through the body suffering from diabetes. Diabetes mellitus is characterized by an excess of sugar in the blood and/or urine. Under the influence of the hormone insulin, which is of vital necessity and which is formed in the pancreas, sugar is converted into heat and muscle power. Insulin regulates the level of sugar in the blood and assists in utilizing and storing the glucose in the body. If too little insulin is formed in the body, the body is unable to adequately utilize sugar and consequently the sugar content of the blood rises. The excess sugar is excreted in the urine. Diabetes is thus a condition that develops due to inability of the body to make appropriate use of the foods as a result of insufficient insulin.

Diabetes can be classified into two groups namely, Type I and Type II. The Type I is insulin dependant diabetes mellitus (IDDM). In this type the pancreas produces little or no insulin; such patients become dependant on outside sources of insulin to control sugar level. This type is common among children. About 5% of the children of diabetics may develop this type of diabetes mellitus. It can be controlled with insulin, proper diet, exercise and careful monitoring.

Type II is non-insulin dependant diabetes mellitus (NIDDM). In this type additional outside insulin is not usually required to sustain life. The body produces some, or at times excessive insulin in its pancreas, but insulin is either not enough for proper functioning or is not being produced quickly enough to influence glucose levels in the blood affectively. So, in many cases, despite high insulin these diabetics have raised blood glucose. The reason is malfunctioning of or defect at the level of muscle cells or adipose — i.e., fat forming tissues which do not adequately respond to insulin for storing glucose in your body cells as a source of energy. The result is again the same the excess of sugar/ glucose in your blood and/ or urine.

Type II is very common among adults and is more common than Type I. This type of diabetes usually occurs in middle or older age and frequently in overweight people. However, this type is less severe than Type I and starts more slowly. Type II is strongly associated with heredity. If both the parents are diabetics there are 25% chances of their children eventually becoming diabetics. The chances of a twin developing diabetes is 100% if one of the two has it. Most often it can be controlled by diet alone, or by a combination of diet, exercise and oral medication.

However, the diabetes that starts in childhood or adolescence is usually more severe than that beginning in middle or old age.

Diabetes has significant impact on the quality of life. Approximately 30 million people in India suffer from it. It is estimated that for every known diabetic, there is a diabetic yet to be discovered. Though any age group can develop diabetes usually this disease is very commonly found among those who are around 35-40 years and overweight. The disease is associated with long term complications involving almost all vital organs like heart, kidneys, eyes and the nervous system. The complications occur earlier in those diabetics when the disease is not adequately controlled. A patient's participation in the treatment goes a long way in averting these long term complications — thus, achieving a better quality of life.

The diabetic may develop symptoms like excessive urination or passing more urine at night, excessive thirst, weight loss and weakness. These symptoms may develop gradually over months or more abruptly within days. Occasionally patients may be brought to hospital in sudden diabetic coma. Unless recognised and treated immediately the outcome may be fatal. Other symptoms such as tingling, numbness, calf muscle pain, frequent skin infections with candida — i.e., the fungus that inhabit vagina and alimentary tract or pus forming organisms may herald the disease. These early symptoms should not be ignored.

Besides patient's education in drugs, diet and exercise have significant contribution in proper management of diabetes. Dietary control, changes and adaptations are important in the treatment of all types and severity of diabetes. This book tells you how diet can help lose weight and improve the action of insulin to achieve ideal body weight over a period of time.

Exercise can be beneficial in reducing the insulin requirement. However, unaccustomed exercise should be avoided by a diabetic on insulin treatment, as hypoglycemic attack — i.e., glucose deficiency in blood may get precipitated. The drugs such as sulfonylureas, which includes tolbutamide, glibenclamide and glipizide, and biguanides which includes matformin and phenformin are in use in our country. These drugs are conveniently recommended to the obese, non-insulin dependent diabetic (NIDDM) patient, in whom it is possible to achieve better control over blood glucose. However, optimum control is rarely achieved without insulin in severe non-insulin dependant diabetic (NIDDM) patients. A physician should be consulted for readjustment of insulin dosage if glucose deficiency in blood occurs.

Anyone who is either a diabetic or has someone diabetic in the family, will find this book very useful and informative in getting acquainted with the disease and by following the guidelines for daily life so that they can — despite the disease and by avoiding the late complications — live a normal life. The chapters on self-control through diet, exercise, self-monitoring, drugs and medication etc. will help the diabetics to make healthier lifestyle adjustments. I am sure this comprehensive book on diabetes written in a very simple and easy language will be of great advantage to the patients, health conscious families, the students and professionals alike.

Dr. SNA Rizvi,

MBBS, MD, FAIID, FIAMS, FISN, FICAI, FICN
Prof. of Medicine
Head of Nephrology and Rheumatology Division
MAMC & Associated LNJP,
GB Pant & Guru Teg Bahadur Eye Hospitals;
Secretary, Diabetic Association of India
(Delhi Branch).

Foreword

During almost 35 years of practice in the field of diabetology I have seen many changes in the philosophy of care for the disease called *diabetes*. Almost all experts in the field now view normal physiological control and good health as essentials in altering the progression of this disease. With newer methods of control has come the necessity for more involvement by patients in their own care. As we recognize the advantages of close control over your diabetes we also recognize the necessity for you to have a thorough understanding of your disease so that you can help yourself to better health.

Ada P. Kahn's emphasis on you as an individual, dealing with your own diabetes, is an important feature of this book. She repeatedly underscores the importance of close communication with your health care team, an essential aspect of modern diabetes management. She also presents up-to-date information clearly enough to help many people better understand their disease. And, finally, the author provides fundamental explanations for most of the everyday problems of living with diabetes in a readable format.

Diabetes is not a disease of the blood sugar alone. Like no other disease, diabetes involves your entire body, from your mind to all organ systems. Therefore, controlling not only your blood sugar, but the factors controlling your blood sugar as well, is important. The body is a complex machine that works best when we have a basic understanding of all of its parts and coordinate their functions. This is especially true in cases of diabetes. In this book, therefore, you will learn about the many aspects of diabetes and its treatment so that you can form an understanding of how it affects your whole body.

Of all the patients I have seen over the years, the individuals who have lived well with the fewest complications and the best control have been those who centered their active lifestyles around good health habits and dietary control as well as proper insulin therapy and a general reduction of high risk factors for disease. These people have helped me recognize that it isn't only the disease itself that contributes to complications; rather, it is the ability of each patient to accept the discipline of living with diabetes in the most compatible way that helps prevent such complications.

Although controlling your diabetes on a day-to-day basis can require a lot of self-discipline, keep in mind that it is still most likely a better fate than having a disease that cannot be treated. Diabetes is a very personal disease, so you will want to gain the best possible understanding of how you can live with it. After all, how you do choose to live with diabetes is up to you and your support team. And while you are learning to manage it well the scientific community is working actively to try to improve treatments.

At this time, I believe that we are making significant advances in understanding, treatment, and care of diabetes. Never before has there been greater hope for normalizing and improving the quality of care. As the researchers seek a complete cure, I believe that you should keep yourself in the best medical state possible so that when better management or a possible cure does come along, you will be more receptive to the latest modes of treatment.

The notable Dr. Joslin, founder of the Joslin Clinic of Boston, frequently emphasized that for many patients diabetes prolonged life. They improved their basic diet and care with the cooperation of their medical advisors and reduced many of the problems they might have had without the self-discipline imposed by diabetes.

Having diabetes, because it requires positive intervention in your good health program, may urge you to reduce weight, stop smoking, get more exercise, and lead an overall healthier lifestyle—benefits you might never have tried to achieve if you didn't have diabetes. At first some interventions may seem like restrictions, but you will soon find that your body responds well to this type of planning for good health.

Planning for good health involves continuing education in your disease. In reviewing books for my diabetic patients to read I find that no references touch all bases. Nor does this book; it was not intended to be an encyclopedia of diabetic care. I consider this book a good starting point for you if you have just been told that you have diabetes as well as if you have had diabetes for a long time and wish to begin your learning process anew. However, knowledge about diabetes changes rapidly. By the time any book is published there are variances in what is recommended in treatment and care. Should what you read in this book differ from what you have learned from your personal health care team, discuss these discrepancies, which may result from personal, individual factors, with them. They know you and your diabetes best.

Your personal physician will outline a treatment plan for you. Your health care team will help you follow that plan. The most important factor in controlling your diabetes, however, is *you*. Help yourself to health. With diabetes you usually have a choice.

Melvin M. Chertack, MD, FACD

Contents

Introduction

If you have been told that you have diabetes, you probably have many questions about how to care for yourself, how your physician will care for you, and whether you can expect to lead a normal life with the disease.

This is an introductory handbook that will teach you some basics about the disease so that you can immediately start to control it and to work with your physician's instructions in optimal ways. If you are the spouse or parent of one who has been diagnosed as having diabetes, this handbook will provide many helpful hints and valuable information with which you can help someone you love lead a more normal, productive, and happy life.

Although this book is not intended to be a complete encyclopedia of information on diabetes, it will give you additional facts about the disease and important guidelines for daily living with diabetes. It is important that you learn as much as you can about diabetes. Some diseases can be treated and controlled just by regularly taking prescription medication. Diabetes is different; it requires somewhat more cooperation and active participation on your part. For example, controlling diabetes may require that you pay serious attention to your eating habits and their regularity, that you change your smoking and drinking habits, lose weight, exercise more, and perhaps use an injected or oral treatment.

Additionally, if you are a female of childbearing age, you will have to pay careful attention to the possibility of becoming pregnant and receive special care during your pregnancy to help assure you of delivering a healthy infant.

Your physician and health care team will provide instructions for you regarding good habits for daily living, continuing to enjoy family life, and buying your health care products economically. However, those in health education recognize that repeated explanations are often needed to supplement a teaching program at the outset of diabetes. And for those who have had diabetes for longer periods of time, frequent reminders are often necessary and important. With these needs in mind, this book has been written to reinforce what you may have learned before.

You may have forgotten to ask some questions during your initial training. You may find some information in this book to think about until your next visit. Or, because you may not have been mentally receptive to what you learned during your earlier education, this book will help you build on what you heard and help you understand better your health care team's recommendations for your personal care.

Therapy for diabetes is highly individualized and requires constant renewing and altering of your care plan as your condition changes. You may find differences between some of the material in this book and what you have learned, but remember that *your* diabetes is managed by you and *your* health care team. Many other sources of information may prove to be helpful to you in understanding your diabetes, but before making any changes in your health care routine you must discuss them with your physician, nutritionist, and other members of your health care team. Again, they know you best.

The diagnosis of diabetes may have been surprising and perhaps even frightening at first. You may have asked, "Why me?" Why should yours be the one of every four families affected by diabetes? Why are you the one out of every 20 people who has diabetes? There are no good answers to these questions. The only answer scientists can give is that they just aren't sure why diabetes affects some people and not others. They *are* sure, however, that many others with diabetes have learned to control their disease and live normal, productive, and happy lives. You can do so, too.

Advances in patient care have greatly improved the quality of life for those with diabetes. The future looks good. However, controlling diabetes will work for you only with your cooperation and participation. You will need patience and understanding while learning to follow your health care team's outline for therapy. Those who care about you will want to augment your therapy with love and encouragement. With more knowledge you can make your personal therapy plan more convenient and more effective. This book can help you do that.

In the following chapters you will learn about some of the things your doctor may do to treat your disease, how you can control your diabetes with diet, medication, and exercise, and what you can do at home to monitor your condition. You will also learn about the special concerns of women and children with diabetes, how to live a full and productive life with diabetes, the price you pay for the disease, and what's ahead in research. Finally, resources for those with diabetes are included so that you can select menu plans, books, organizations, and other sources of special assistance in your community. A glossary is included to give you a working knowledge of the vocabulary of diabetes and to help you explain the disease and its treatment to a child, an elderly person, or someone else about whom you care.

As you learn to care for yourself and follow your physician's instructions, this book can help you help yourself to health.

1
Getting Acquainted with Diabetes

Getting acquainted with anything or anyone usually means asking questions, seeking answers, and thinking about new ideas. When you get a new car, for example, you want to know how everything works. Sometimes you want to know *why* things work the way they do and what to do in case they don't work correctly.

Because your health is such a personal matter, you will have even more questions when you are getting acquainted with a disease. And, if you have lived with a disease for a long time, continued learning about—or reacquainting yourself with—the disease is an ongoing process.

If you are getting acquainted or reacquainted with diabetes, you will want to know what diabetes is all about and how you can successfully incorporate treatment for the disease into your lifestyle. In this chapter you will learn about what diabetes is, whether symptoms are always noticeable, what may cause diabetes, how diabetes can be controlled and why it is important to control it, what diet and menu planning will mean for you, and what those with insulin-dependent diabetes and non-insulin-dependent diabetes should know.

You may already know that there are two names for diabetes:

diabetes mellitus and *diabetes insipidus*. The term *diabetes melli-tus* was derived from the Greek words meaning *passing through* and *sweet as honey*. Diabetes mellitus is a condition characterized by an excess of sugar in the blood and/or urine. Diabetes insipi-dus is characterized by an excess of fluid loss by the body. In this book the word *diabetes* is used throughout and refers to *diabetes mellitus*, the disease you may have heard people refer to as "too much sugar."

What is Diabetes?

Diabetes is a disease that develops due to your body's inability to make appropriate use of the foods you eat as a result of insufficient insulin.

Normally the food you eat is converted within your body into a form of sugar called *glucose*, which your cells use as a source of energy. Glucose causes an increase in your blood glucose level, which in turn signals the release of a hormone called *insulin* from the islet cells (the cluster of cells in the pancreas known as islets of Langerhans) of the pancreas, a gland in the abdomen. Insulin regulates the level of glucose in your blood and assists in utilizing and storing glucose in your body.

All human beings need insulin. Most people have enough. If you have diabetes, however, you may produce none at all or perhaps just not enough to help the glucose from your blood transfer to the appropriate cells. Without insulin, glucose isn't used by your cells and thus builds up in your blood.

Diabetes is not contagious. There is no cure for it at this time. However, the disease *can* be controlled. This book will help you understand how to control your diabetes and the importance of doing so.

Different Types of Diabetes

Not all cases of diabetes are alike. Your case may be distinctly different from your neighbor's or friend's.

There are several types of diabetes. Within these types the course of the disease varies. The following classification system for diabetes was endorsed by the board of directors of the American Diabetes Association at its 1979 annual meeting.

Type I

Type I is insulin-dependent diabetes, and it can occur at any age, though it most commonly occurs during youth. This type of diabetes used to be known as *juvenile-onset diabetes* and is still called that by some physicians and health care professionals. About one of every 2,500 children has this disease. Because the pancreas produces little or no insulin, such patients become dependent on outside sources of insulin. Before the discovery of insulin in 1921 children with insulin-dependent diabetes had a short life expectancy. Now the disease can be controlled with insulin, proper diet and exercise, and careful monitoring.

Type II

Type II is non-insulin-dependent diabetes; additional insulin is not usually required to sustain life. The American Diabetes Association further divides this category into subtypes that include obese non-insulin-dependent diabetes and nonobese non-insulin-dependent diabetes. (Estimates are that 60–90 percent of those with non-insulin-dependent diabetes in western societies are obese.) Non-insulin-dependent diabetes used to be called *maturity-onset diabetes* and may still be called that by some health care professionals. Type II diabetes is much more common than Type I. If you have non-insulin-dependent diabetes, you are one of 5 million Americans with the disease. This type is less severe than insulin-dependent diabetes and starts more slowly.

While patients with this type of diabetes produce some, or at times even excessive, insulin in their pancreas, it either is not enough for proper function or is not being produced quickly enough to influence glucose levels in the blood effectively. This type of the disease usually occurs in middle or older age and frequently in overweight people. It can most often be controlled by diet alone or by a combination of diet, exercise, and oral medication.

Table 1
Characteristic of Insulin-Dependent and
Non-Insulin-Dependent Diabetes

	Insulin-Dependent (Type I)	Non-Insulin-Dependent (Type II)
Age of onset	Usually during youth, but can occur at any age.	Usually during adulthood; more common in older people.
How noticed	Usually appears abruptly and progresses rapidly.	Gradual in onset; the disease may go unnoticed for years.
Family background	Diabetes not always present in other family members.	Often diabetes was present in other members of the family.
Treatment	Insulin injections are necessary. Diet, exercise, and emotional control are necessary.	Insulin injections are not always necessary. Oral medications are sometimes recommended. Diet, exercise, and emotional control are necessary.
Complications	Problems affecting blood vessels, eyes, kidneys, and nerves may occur at any age.	Problems affecting blood vessels, eyes, kidneys, and nerves may occur at any age.
Linked to obesity	Not necessarily.	80 percent of all patients are overweight at time of diagnosis.

Impaired Glucose Tolerance

Until recently the terms *borderline, chemical,* and *latent diabetes* were used to refer to this condition. Now, according to recommendations by the American Diabetes Association, the term *impaired glucose tolerance* refers to the condition in which fasting plasma glucose level is normal but after glucose intake the levels are abnormally elevated. You'll read more about this condition in Chapter 2, which describes in more detail the types of tests your physician will do to diagnose and monitor your diabetes.

Gestational Diabetes

The term *gestational diabetes* is used only to refer to diabetes that develops during pregnancy. You'll read more about this in Chapter 6, which explains the special concerns of women with diabetes in more detail.

Other Types

There are also many types of diabetes associated with certain conditions and syndromes, such as diabetes induced by drugs or chemicals, diabetes secondary to pancreatic disease, and diabetes secondary to endocrine disease. These types are not discussed in this book as they occur less frequently.

What Causes Diabetes?

Although the causes of diabetes are still unknown, medical science does know that certain factors contribute to its development. One factor is heredity. You may have a tendency to develop diabetes because other members of your family have it. A child of nondiabetics *can* become diabetic, however, since the disease may skip generations because of genetic coding that prevents it from appearing in every generation. Stresses that affect the cells of the body seem to set the stage for diabetes in these people. One such stress is extra weight. Obesity, affecting insulin utilization, contributes to diabetes. Researchers estimate that 80 percent of the people with diabetes are also overweight at the time they are diagnosed as having diabetes.

Stresses can be emotional or physical, such as surgery or a serious infection, an accident, or emotional shock. Many medications affect the body in a stressful way. Pregnancy also places extra stresses on the body, and diabetes is often diagnosed in pregnant women or women who have repeated miscarriages.

People who develop diabetes, especially Type II, frequently also have high blood pressure; people of middle or old age are more likely to develop diabetes than younger people, and women are more likely to have diabetes than men.

Diabetic Symptoms

About the time you were told that you had diabetes you may have noticed increased thirst, excessive urination, increased appetite and loss of weight, or itchy skin. You may also have noticed sores and cuts healed slowly, that you tired easily and became drowsy often, or that you had impaired vision (see Table 1-2). In the early stages of the disease, however, many people do not notice any symptoms. Many older adults who have diabetes have no symptoms other than a vague feeling of not being well. In such persons the disease is detected through a blood sugar test. Your physician may have suspected that you have diabetes by detecting glucose in your urine. The diagnosis may have been confirmed with further tests.

Table 2
Diabetes Symtoms*

Type I	*Type II*
Frequent urination	Excess weight
Increased thirst	Drowsiness
Unusual hunger	Blurred vision
Weight loss	Tingling and numbness in hands and feet
Irritability	Skin infections
Weakness and fatigue	Slow healing of cuts (especially on the feet)
Nausea and vomiting	Itching

*Source : American Diabetic Association

Controlling Diabetes

Diabetes can be controlled through effective management of the balance of sugar (or glucose) and insulin, to enable your body to function well. Your physician and health care team will tailor an individualized therapy routine to your needs. This may include special attention to your diet, a plan for exercise, and possibly medication in the form of injections of insulin or pills to be taken orally. The diet plan will help you control your intake of food as well as your weight. The amount of exercise you do will determine the rate at which your body demands sugar to produce energy, and insulin will regulate how fast and effectively the sugar is used to meet your needs for energy.

Why is it Important to Control Diabetes As Soon As it is Detected?

As soon as your diabetes is detected it is important that you immediately begin a program to control the disease. The aim of your treatment plan will be to restore the balance of sugar and insulin in your body and to prevent and relieve symptoms. You can do this through diet, exercise, and blood sugar–reducing medications and, most important, by understanding the disease, its complications, and its treatment.

A properly treated person with diabetes can be free of symptoms and feel well. Without adequate medical treatment, however, symptoms may appear or increase in severity. For example, in many people with diabetes complications occur in blood vessels. Because diabetics are more prone to problems with blood vessels, such conditions appear earlier and advance more rapidly than in nondiabetics. And since both the large and small blood vessels can be involved, complications, such as hypertension and atherosclerosis, often are the principal problems in the care of diabetics. While the mechanism of diabetic disease of the blood vessels is not clearly identified, it is also known that vascular disease (disease of the blood vessels) may not be as prevalent or proceeds more slowly in those with well-controlled diabetes than in those in whom the disease is poorly controlled.

Vascular disease causes other complications of the circulatory system, including heart attacks. Diabetic women, especially after menopause, have more heart disease than women who do not have diabetes. Also, because of changes in the arteries due to diabetes, some diabetics have peripheral circulatory disturbances, especially in their legs.

Diabetics have more kidney disease than nondiabetics. This occurs because blood vessels serving the kidneys often are affected, and recurrent infections of the urinary tract can be more common.

Vascular changes also can affect the eyes where blood vessels are very tiny and fragile. The fact that diabetes is the leading cause of blindness emphasizes the need for preserving this important faculty.

Neuropathy (damage to the neural pathways) may be another long-term complication of diabetes. The most common form affects the legs and may cause numbness, tingling, and sometimes severe pain. Other nerve pathways can be affected as well. Diabetics' feet are vulnerable to any kind of injury, and foot care is extremely important. Joint and skeletal muscle problems are also affected by diabetes, as is the gastrointestinal tract.

To prevent these and other complications it is essential that you begin a treatment plan as soon as possible after your diabetes is diagnosed. An important part of your treatment will be your diet.

Paying Attention to Diet

Your doctor will determine the meal plan that is best for you, based on your age, weight, activity level, occupation, and other medical requirements. You will be responsible for controlling the amount of sugar that gets into your bloodstream by controlling the kind and amount of food you eat.

While your diet may be "special" in the sense that you now will pay more attention to it than you did in the past, you are very likely to continue to eat the same foods as nondiabetics should eat. The main difference will be in being sure to eat at the right time and to eat the amounts recommended by your doctor. Your doctor will tell you about a food exchange system that will enable you to have flexibility and normal food within your diet. By following the food exchange system you can trade, for example, an ounce of meat for a portion of cheese or an egg. There are many foods you can have without any restriction at all, such as many low-calorie vegetables, fat-free bouillon and broth, and decaffeinated coffee, and tea in moderation.

You won't need any special equipment for your kitchen, other than a standard eight-ounce measuring cup, a measuring teaspoon and tablespoon, and a small scale. Recommendations for your meals usually will be stated in terms of cups, tablespoons, and teaspoons. Sometimes a few weight measurements will be recommended. You will learn more about watching weights and measures of foods, calories, and sugar content in Chapter 4.

Menu Planning

Menu planning will be an important part of your lifestyle with diabetes. If you have insulin-dependent diabetes, you will have to plan when and how much to eat so that meals and snacks coincide with the effects and timing of your daily insulin injections. You will also have to consume a specific number of calories to feel well and maintain ideal weight and a more normal blood-sugar level. If your health care team recommends that you control your blood sugar level with diet and/or oral medication, you will be asked to follow a more regular, calculated meal plan to maintain normal weight and avoid sharp variations in your blood sugar. If you are overweight, you can use the plan as a weight-loss diet to achieve a more normal weight. Normal weight is important because excessive fat cells interfere with your body's use of insulin.

What Those with Insulin-Dependent Diabetes Should Know?

With insulin-dependent diabetes, when insulin injections begin your symptoms may disappear and the disease may go into a stage of remission or temporarily appear inactive. In this phase your pancreas will again secrete insulin. Your need for extra insulin may decrease or disappear. The remission phase frequently lasts as long as two or more years, and during this period it may be hard to believe that you have the disease. Your blood sugar level may remain within a normal range. Without explanation your blood sugar may go up again and again create the need for additional amounts of insulin.

During the remission phase a well-balanced diet will be very important. If possible, you should try to maintain your ideal weight. However, the remission phase may end or may not occur at all. When this happens your diabetes may be less stable, your pancreas will secrete varying amounts of insulin, and your condition may develop into what is known as *brittle* or poorly controlled diabetes because your blood sugar may fluctuate widely during the same day for no apparent reason. *Brittle* is simply the term some physicians use for a markedly fluctuating blood sugar level. In this stage it usually indicates poor daily management, and insulin, exercise, or activity may affect your blood sugar level. Better regulation of your diabetes may be necessary through dietary means, additional exercise, and alteration of your insulin intake. Close regulation may be a greater problem if you have little or no insulin production of your own.

Two Medical Emergencies to Know About

If you have insulin-dependent diabetes, you can avoid two medical emergencies by carefully monitoring your blood sugar level. Ketoacidosis (diabetic coma) is a condition of elevated blood sugar and breakdown of muscle and fat that results in a disturbance in the acid-alkaline balance in your body and causes loss of consciousness or coma. Diabetic coma can occur because of a lack of the necessary insulin dose in the presence of the effects of stress (physicial or emotional), infection, or major illness. Recognition of symptoms and prompt treatment by a physician are important. Symptoms may include flushed, dry skin, drowsiness, a fruity breath odor, deep labored breathing, vomiting, and abdominal pain.

Hypoglycemia (low blood sugar) is a condition that can occur because of an excess of insulin, too much exercise, or not enough food. Fortunately most cases of hypoglycemia are easily reversible. You can avoid this unpleasant complication by understanding how insulin, food, and exercise interact. Further, you can use urine testing or blood sugar testing as a guide in controlling your blood sugar. While many people with insulin-dependent diabetes seldom develop this complication, it is a frequent and disturbing one that requires knowledge of diabetes and cooperation with your health care team.

What Those with Non-Insulin-Dependent Diabetes Should Know

It is possible that you had subtle symptoms of diabetes for years and did not know that you had the disease. Weight gain, increased thirst, and fatigue may have been building up over a number of years. Because the disease has been present for a long time, you may have some complications at the time a diagnosis is made. These might include hypertension (high blood pressure), heart disease, vascular disease (small blood vessel disease), or kidney disease. Your physician will treat these problems along with your diabetes. It is important to treat such complications as early as possible because a combination of high blood pressure, diabetes, and kidney disease is a triple threat to your good health. You'll learn why in Chapter 10.

Many people, however, do not have any complications and can take actions recommended by their physicians concerning diet, exercise, medication in the form of pills instead of insulin injection, and good mental health. If you have non-insulin-dependent diabetes, it is possible that your diabetes may reverse itself and that your blood sugar levels may return to normal and stay that way, particularly if you maintain good diet and exercise habits.

Good diet, ideal weight, adequate exercise, adequate insulin availability, and a stable mental attitude are the keys to treatment for diabetes.

2
Diagnosing and Monitoring Diabetes

Your physician may have suspected that you have diabetes because of a high sugar (glucose) level found in your blood or urine during a routine office visit. At the time you may not have noticed any symptoms. Many diabetics, however, do notice symptoms—including excessive urination, unusual thirst, weight loss despite good appetite, or constant fatigue—and seek medical advice because of them.

Detecting High Glucose and Ketones

When adequately distributed throughout your body, glucose gives you energy. If the glucose level in your blood or urine is high, it means that the glucose is not being channeled properly. This happens when too little of the hormone insulin is produced or when the insulin that is produced is not used appropriately by the body.

Insulin is responsible for clearing sugar out of your bloodstream and getting it into cells, where it is used or stored. In a diabetic, because enough insulin isn't there or isn't working properly, glucose just accumulates in the blood. After a certain point the blood glucose becomes so high that the kidneys, which filter waste products from the blood, begin to overflow some of the glucose into the urine. Your physician can measure your glucose level through several tests using urine and blood specimens.

In addition to measuring the glucose level, urine and blood tests can indicate the presence of ketones. Without insulin, fat stores in the body break down and substances called *ketones, ketone bodies,* or *acetone* are produced. Because of their acidic nature, ketones can lead to complications when they accumulate in the blood. At high enough levels ketones overflow into the urine.

Glucose and ketone levels in the urine and blood may be high because of stress as well as a low insulin level. A finding of high levels of glucose or ketones indicates to your physician that further investigation is necessary.

Urine Tests

Urine testing is part of most physicians' routines in giving complete physical examinations. Urine tests are basic diagnostic tools that can give physicians valuable information about how your body is working.

In a form of urine testing known as *semiquantitative* your doctor may use either a tablet or one of several brands of paper or plastic strips to determine the approximate sugar or ketone level in your urine. Only a small sample of urine is needed, and the test takes only a few seconds. The paper or plastic strips are coated with chemicals that change colors according to sugar and ketone concentration. For example, one type of strip ranges from yellow through green to dark blue. With this test a color closer to dark blue indicates a high concentration of sugar in the urine. However, if you are taking certain medications, aspirin, or vitamin C, these substances may interfere with the dyes on the strips and distort the readings. Your physician will ask you about medications you are taking so that test results can be interpreted properly.

An advantage of semiquantitative urine testing is that it is fast and can be done easily by your doctor. The disadvantage of urine tests, in general, however, is that they are less accurate and harder to interpret than blood tests. Because the point at which your kidneys begin to spill glucose into your urine may differ from the point in other people, urine test readings may not always accurately reflect the level of glucose in your blood.

Another urine test your physician may do is known as a *quantitative* measurement in a timed sample. This test might be ordered by your physician after a high or low reading has been found with a semiquantitative test. One advantage of this type of test is that only glucose and ketones are measured, and other chemicals in your blood that might have caused false higher or lower readings with the chemically coated paper strips used in semiquantitative testing are removed. Another advantage is that the exact concentration, rather than a range, of glucose and ketones in the urine is measured.

Because the urine must be collected very accurately in such tests, (whereas only a small sample is necessary for the semiquantitative tests), it is inconvenient. If the physician orders a 24-hour sample, this means that all urine during that period must be collected and brought to the laboratory. Another disadvantage is that, depending on the point at which the patient's kidneys actually begin to spill sugar and ketones into the urine, this may or may not be an accurate reflection of glucose levels.

Blood Tests

Blood glucose tests are also used to indicate whether or not you have too much or not enough sugar in your blood and whether or not ketones are present. If you are curious about the numbers you hear or read, ask your doctor to explain your test results to you. Comparing blood test results with others, however, is not a good idea, because different blood tests yield different results.

The easiest and fastest procedure for measuring glucose and ketones in the blood is to use plastic or paper strips like those used in urine tests. These strips give a range, not an exact value. Other methods, called *reagent kits* and *rapid analytical systems*, are also used by many physicians. These tests use chemicals to test blood samples in a rapid single-step process.

Which is Better?
Urine-Sugar or Blood-Sugar Test

- Urine or blood sugar tests are the commonest test performed to know the state of diabetic control.

- Blood contains some amount of sugar (80 to 140 mg%) round the clock, since certain tissues like brain cannot survive without readily available glucose.

- When the blood sugar exceeds, 180 mg% sugar appears in urine. **Urine test is only a rough guide,** e.g. if there is no sugar in urine it can only mean that blood sugar at that time is less than180 mg% (it can be anything 60 to 180 mg%). Urine sugar approximates with blood sugar in the ways mentioned below.

Urine Sugar	Blood Sugar mg%
+	200
+ +	250
+ + +	300
+ + + +	350

(Urine Sugar values bracketed together $=$ Blood Sugar values)

- Since urine is secreted drop by drop by the kidney and stored in bladder to be evacuated at longer intervals, if we wish to correlate unine sugar with blood sugar level we must test second sample of urine—i.e. evacuate the bladder, dicard it and pass urine after half an hour, test that sample. It will give better idea of blood sugar level at that time.

- **Blood sugar is more accurate parameter for assessing control of diabetes**

Blood glucose concentration is one of the best measurements of the presence of diabetes as well as diabetic control. But, because this test measures the blood glucose level at only one instant, it may not represent your usual condition. For example, a trip to your doctor's office can cause stress that can result in an abnormally high glucose value. Blood sugar is affected by the food eaten, the amount of time after or before eating, and activity and stress. A sample taken within two hours after you have eaten gives the most sensitive results after a measured glucose intake. Evaluating your fasting or before glucose intake level indicates the extent to which carbohydrates from your last meal have been removed from your bloodstream. The fasting glucose concentration is the measure of blood sugar after a lack of intake for more than four hours or overnight. If you have diabetes, your glucose concentration is usually lowest in this state.

Glycosylated Hemoglobin

Another blood test your physician may perform to learn more about the glucose concentration in your blood involves glycosylated hemoglobin. *Glycosylated hemoglobin* is created when glucose is attached to hemoglobin cells (red blood cells). The concentration of these glycosylated hemoglobin molecules is a good barometer of average glucose content, as it is higher in diabetics than in nondiabetics. It is also very high in patients who poorly control their diabetes.

Glucose attaches to the hemoglobin slowly, depending on the concentration of glucose in the blood. Since the life span of a red blood cells is about four months, a high concentration of glycosylated hemoglobin in your blood indicates that the condition has been building over a period of time. A measurement of glycosylated hemoglobin is like peering back in time. Because this test indicates whan happened previously, rather than what is taking place now, it does help your doctor in terms of establishing or making adjustments in your treatment. Also, the test at present is expensive. However, for long-term monitoring of diabetic control, glycosylated hemoglobin tests are useful, and your physician may make use of them in treating you.

Glucose Tolerance Tests

The basic glucose tolerance test may be ordered by your physician as part of a complete physical examination or specifically because diabetes is suspected. It involves taking a small specimen of blood from a vein in your arm. Over approximately a several-hour period, multiple separate readings of your blood glucose level are taken. These measurements, when plotted on a graph, graphically portray how your body handles glucose. The test is especially valuable because it can confirm the presence of a condition known as *impaired glucose tolerance*. While people who have impaired glucose tolerance do have elevated blood glucose levels after meals, impaired glucose tolerance is not necessarily diabetes, and their fasting blood sugar is normal. However, people who have this condition may be more likely than others to develop active diabetes.

Glucose Concentration Value Chart (mg per ml of blood)	
Normal	
a) Fasting value	065-100
b) 2 hrs. after meals	100-120
Impaired Glucose Tolerance*	
a) Fasting value	105-120
b) 2 hrs. after taking Glucose	120-150
Diabetes Mellitus**	
a) Fasting value	$\geq$120
b) 2 hrs. after taking Glucose	$\geq$180

Source : WHO

* These values are the boarderline cases of mild high blood sugar and can be recommended for further investigations/tests by the doctor so that the person with such condition should take necessary precaution to control it in time.

** $\geq$Stands for equal to and greater than.

If your physician orders a glucose tolerance test, it will be scheduled in the morning after you have had three days of good food intake so that your body can handle sugar optimally. You will be asked not to eat breakfast that morning so that your first blood sample will reflect your fasting glucose level. Next you will be given a beverage or test meal containing glucose to drink or eat. On some occasions glucose is administered intravenously. At various hourly intervals after you have taken the glucose, blood samples will be taken and the glucose level of your blood will be measured.

This test is usually not used by physicians during periods of long dietary restriction, illness, or disability or without the three-day good food intake preparation.

If you do not have diabetes or impaired glucose tolerance, the resulting readings, plotted on a graph, will show a normal pattern. If you *do* have diabetes, the graph will show that your blood glucose level rose and kept rising and did not even begin to drop by the end of the test. If you have impaired glucose tolerance, the graph will look much like the nondiabetic's graph, but it will indicate higher blood sugar concentrations with normal fasting or end-of-test levels. The levels will fall between the range of the nondiabetic and the diabetic on the graph. The term *impaired glucose tolerance* refers to the condition in which the fasting plasma glucose level is between normal and diabetic levels. This term is used instead of the term *borderline, chemical* or *latent* diabetes.

If a glucose tolerance test reveals that you have impaired glucose tolerance, your doctor may recommend that you have further tests. Also, because people with impaired glucose tolerance are more likely to develop diabetes, and because at this stage diabetes is preventable, your doctor may advise you to lose weight, cut your intake of simple sugars, exercise more, and avoid cardiovascular risk factors, including high blood pressure, smoking, and high cholesterol levels.

Steroid Glucose Tolerance Test

The steroid glucose tolerance test is a variation of the glucose tolerance test. A steroid (cortisone) is administered that mimics stress in the body. Psychological stress, obesity, and illness are all factors that may precipitate diabetes. If this test produces results showing impaired glucose tolerance, it is an indication that you may develop diabetes, especially if other members of your family have had diabetes.

A combination of these tests will help your physician diagnosis and monitor your diabetes. Continued reevaluation is necessary because your blood sugar level changes in response to your diet, exercise, medication, and emotional stress. With the aid of testing procedures, your physician can help you control your diabetes.

3
Medical Treatment Tailored for You

Your physician's goal will be to help you maintain a normal blood glucose level and to minimize, whenever possible, possible complications of the disease. While diet is the first line of treatment in non-insulin dependent diabetes, if your blood sugar level cannot be brought under control that way, a blood sugar-lowering therapy will be prescribed for you.

If you have insulin-dependent diabetes, your physician will prescribe insulin in an injectable form or an oral medication as well as a special diet and exercise program to interact with your diet and lifestyle. Your individual case will determine which type of insulin will work best for you. Also, if you have the type of job that makes taking insulin difficult, your physician may try to prescribe oral medication if he or she believes that it will be effective for you. Whether you use injected insulin or oral medication, it is most important that you follow your physician's instructions regarding diet. Physicians say that the greatest error diabetic patients can make is to use therapy to reduce blood sugar and then neglect their diet. The goal of treatment is to preserve your insulin output as much as possible. You can do this by complying with the diet recommended for you, getting your weight down to your ideal level, and taking or injecting your medication as it is prescribed for you.

Understanding Insulin

Insulin prevents or controls many symptoms of diabetes and contributes to your overall strength and weight control. Insulin has become easier and safer to use since 1921 when it was developed. Present-day insulin preparations are purer and more concentrated than those of some years ago, and less fluid is required to obtain the necessary dose. Consequently, diabetics now can have fairly good control over their disease more readily. Also, needles for insulin injections, particularly the disposable type, have been improved and are now small and nearly painless. Overall, insulin therapy has become more convenient and easier than it used to be.

Your doctor will review with you the various types of insulin available, the type and dose that best meets your individual needs, and how and when to take your injection. For example, you may be advised to take the insulin about one-half hour before breakfast or before the evening meal or occasionally before other meals or bedtime.

Where does insulin come from? Most insulin now being used to treat diabetes comes from the pancreases of hogs and cattle. It is manufactured as pure pork insulin or pure beef insulin, though the most widely used insulin is a mixture of both kinds. Your physician will determine which is best for you. Beef and pork insulins are not chemically the same, and they are not chemically the same as insulin made by the human pancreas. All types of insulin are proteins and are made from the body's building blocks called amino acids. Human, beef, and pork insulins all have 51 amino acids. Pork insulin has one amino acid different from human insulin, while beef insulin and human insulin differ in three amino acids. Pork insulin, is more like human insulin.

Recently, human insulan has been produced by bioengineering techniques. It has been cleared by the U.S. Food and Drug Administration and will soon be available for use.

Some people react differently to beef insulin and pork insulin. One person may have an allergic reaction whenever beef insulin is injected while another may not. The same is true of pork insulin.

For individuals who have certain types of adverse reactions to mixed insulin, the more highly purified pork insulin may be the best choice.

If you are not allergic or resistant to any type of insulin, it may not matter which type you use. However, you may have a minor amount of resistance to either type of insulin, which does not become apparent until the type of insulin is changed. For example, if you change from one type to another, you may find that you need more or less of the new type to bring your glucose level untder control.

Your medical team, consisting of your physician, a nurse, and usually a nutritionist, will assist you in understanding how to inject insulin, what to expect in the way of reactions, and how to avoid them. They will discuss with you the importance of rotating the site of injection. For example, you should not use any site of injection more than once every 15 days because doing so may cause the absorption of insulin to vary and fluctuations in blood sugar may occur. Also, rotation of sites helps avoids bumps and indentations in your skin. Insulin is absorbed more slowly in your legs than your abdomen and more slowly in the arms than in your abdomen. Commonly recommended sites are the outer area of the upper arm, the abdominal area below the waist, the upper area of the buttock just behind the hipbone, and the front of the thigh above the knee, as shown below.

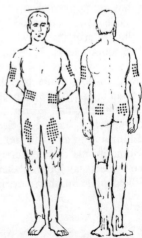

If Your Doctor Has Prescribed Insulin Injections For Treatment

☐ Don't resent or try to escape from it, it is essential for your good health and survivial.

☐ Tablets are no substitute for Insulin. Your diabetes has reached a stage when tablets are not effective.

☐ Insulin is not habit forming. In some cases, once the emergency situation is over you could go back to tablets or diet alone.

☐ Insulin injected works only for 6 to 24 hours. It has to be repeated every day. There is no fixed duration of course of Insulin.

☐ Insulin cannot be given by mouth. You have to accept Insulin injections.

☐ Learn to take Insulin injections yourself.

☐ Learn :
  - How to use and sterilize syringes
  - How to fill the required dose in the syringe
  - How and where to take Insulin injections
  - To manage minor adjustment of dose of Insulin
  - To recognize hypoglycemic reactions and its remedy
  - To check urine or blood sugar yourself

☐ Carry identity card mentioning your name & address, dose of Insulin and address of your family doctor.

Pharmaceutical companies that produce insulin prepare instructional materials that explain techniques for injecting insulin; because these materials are readily available, details are not given here. Also, details on mixing insulin will be given by your physician as well as the manufacturer of the product you will use.

No two people are alike, and an identical dose of insulin in two people may have vastly different effects. That is why your physician will explain the importance of monitoring the effects of the insulin through urine or blood sugar testing.

If your job or exercise routine calls for using certain parts of your body more than others, your physician will give you special instructions regarding injections. For example, if you are a jogger and must move your arms and legs, you will probably be advised not to inject insulin into your thighs and arms because exercise causes more rapid absorption of insulin from the site of the injection. Rapid absorption can lead to hypoglycemia.

Your medical team will tell you how to treat an insulin reaction by yourself. While insulin reactions are not common, they can happen, and you will need to know how to recognize these and take care of yourself. You will probably be advised to carry. carbohydrate and protein sources to eat before you exercise or work strenuously and to keep quick sources of carbohydrates handy, such as sugar-containing fruit drinks, honey, or orange juice. You may want to ask your health care team about using glucagon therapy for insulin shock. Glucagon is a substance produced by the alpha cells of the pancreas which increases blood sugar and reverses an insulin shock reaction.

Oral Medications

In addition to injected insulin, diabetes medication comes in the form of pills known as *oral hypoglycemic agents*, which lower the blood sugar level. They have been used since 1956 when the first of the drugs became available. Because the American Diabetes Association recommends that the basis of treatment in most cases of non-insulin-dependent diabetes should be diet, they say that oral drugs (as well as insulin) should most usually be prescribed only *after* diet therapy alone has failed. At times, however, they can be used as weight reduction is being achieved and medical conditions require blood sugar to be lowered.

Your physician may initially recommend that you use the blood sugar–lowering pills to determine if you can control your disease that way. Along with taking the pills it will be important to follow your diet, exercise, try to remove some of the stressful factors from your life, and monitor your sugar level. This may be effective for patients who are still producing insulin but not enough of it to control their blood sugar without these drugs.

Diabetes pills are *not* oral insulin. While they can significantly reduce the blood sugar level in non-insulin-dependent diabetics, they reduce the blood sugar level only to a small degree in most insulin-dependent diabetics. If the pills are effective, they cause the pancreas to produce extra insulin. The pills work only if the pancreas can still produce insulin. If you are a less severely afflicted non-insulin-dependent diabetic, your physician may prescribe the pills for you. Pills may be prescribed for non-insuln-dependent diabetics whose activities don't permit regular meals or for those whose irregular schedules would interfere with the use of insulin. Some people, such as those with poor vision, have difficulty using syringes and are not given insulin for that reason if sufficient, though less than ideal, control can be achieved. If necessary, a support system involving friends, relatives, neighbors, or your health care team may be developed. Such a system can provide help in working out methods for your treatment.

The various oral medications available have different instructions and different degrees of effectiveness for different people. Some are taken only once a day, and others have to be taken as often as three times a day.

Hypoglycemic reactions are much less frequent with pills because pills work more slowly than injected insulin and are usually less potent. If you take insulin, the blood sugar level goes down, whether or not you eat. With pills the pancreas still produces some insulin as a response to the chemical action within your body. Some researchers say that use of pills makes the body tissues more receptive to the insulin that is produced, and thus the insulin you have is used more efficiently.

Another advantage of pills is that you will be less hungry than with injected insulin, because while your blood sugar won't drop as low or as fast, your appetite won't be stimulated as much.

If you take oral medication for diabetes, it is important to know that these pills may interact unfavorably with some other medications. For example, aspirin and some prescription drugs intensify the effects of diabetes pills. Additionally, you should know that some drugs, such as diuretics, steroids, nicotinic acids, and birth control pills may interfere with the effectiveness of diabetes pills. That's why it is essential that you tell your physician that you are taking other medications if you are advised to take a medication for your diabetes.

Generic Drugs

To avoid the high cost of regular drug use, many people prefer to switch to generic drugs. Only two commonly prescribed oral antidiabetic drugs are available generically: tolbutamide and chlorpropamide. While many generic drugs are safe, the Food and Drug Administration says that these generics may not be as effective as the nongeneric items. Batches of the generic drugs have been recalled, while in 22 or more years of production none of the nongeneric antidiabetic drugs have been recalled.

Generic antidiabetic drugs can be harmful if they work too quickly or strongly, because a hypoglycemic (low blood sugar) reaction may occur. Also, if the drug isn't as strong as it should be, your blood sugar level may become elevated without warning. If you want to switch from one brand to another, do so only under your physician's supervision. If your diabetes is stabilized with one particular product, you might jeopardize that control by switching to one to which your system reacts differently, advises the American Diabetes Association.

Use of generics in control of diabetes requires caution. Making an unmonitored switch from a prescribed brand to a generic may mean loss of diabetes control. In that case your cost in additional medical attention may more than outweigh any savings realized from purchasing the generic products.

Because some generic products cost less than their prescription equivalents, many physicians write prescriptions for the generic drugs. If your physician thinks a generic drug will work well for you, he or she will so indicate on your prescription.

Whether you use injected insulin or an oral medication, it will be regular use of the preparation, plus diet, a regular exercise program, and a good mental outlook, that will help control your disease. Medication alone won't do the job. The combined treatment approach works best.

Table 3

How to Indentify a Diabetic Emergency*

	Low blood sugar (Hypoglycemia)	High blood sugar (Hyperglycemia with Acidosis)
Onset	Sudden	Gradual
Signs	Staggering, poor coordination Anger, bad temper. Pale color Confusion, disorientation Sudden hunger Sweating Eventual stupor or unconsciousness	Drowsiness Extreme thirst Very frequent urination Flushed skin Vomiting Fruity or wine-like odor on breath Heavy breathing Eventual stupor or unconsciousness
Causes	Failure to eat before strenuous exercise; delayed or missed meals.	Undiagnosed diabetes. Insulin not taken. Stress, illness, or injury. Too much food, drink, or both.
What to Do	Provide sugar. If the person can swallow without choking, offer any food such as soft drinks, fruit juice, candy. Do not use diet drinks when blood sugar is low. If the person does not feel better in 10–15 minutes, take	If you are uncertain about whether the person is suffering from high blood sugar or low blood sugar, give him or her some food or drink that contains some sugar. If there is no response in 10–15 minutes, the person needs medical attention. Do not give any food or drink if the person is unable to swallow. Call

*Source : American Diabetic Association

4
Self-Control
Through Diet

Diet is one line of treatment that is very important to the control of your diabetes.

Diet does not necessarily mean eating less; it means planning your meals so that you get the nutrients you require at the proper time and maintain your ideal weight. Your diet can help you lose weight and improve the action of insulin. At the same time your diet can help reduce the risk of cardiovascular disease. Proper diet also calls for increasing your fiber intake, an important factor in the control of diabetes. While diet can do all of these things, in many ways it is no different from a nondiabetic's ideal diet—ideal weight, health, and nutritional balance are all maintained.

Your Dietary History

Before recommending a diet for you, your health care team will take your dietary history. This information will make them familiar with your eating habits and will enable them to assess your current nutritional state and select foods for your diet. Your physician and nutritionist may ask you many questions: Where do you eat? How fast? Who prepares your food? Why do you eat? What are your ethnic food preferences? What is your budget? When do you eat? Whom do you eat with? How much do you know about nutrition? Do you have storage facilities for food?

How many family members are there in your household? Do you eat while you watch TV?

Your physician may also ask you to keep a diary of your eating habits and your schedule. All of this information is important because it provides details with which a diet can be tailored to your lifestyle. In addition to prescribing a diet for you, your health care team will also follow through to be sure that you understand the nutritional principles underlying your individualized diet.

Food is Your Fuel

Your diet provides you with nutrients such as vitamins and minerals, as well as fats, carbohydrates, and proteins—the three major energy sources in all foods. The most common carbohydrates are sugars and starches. In addition to yielding energy, proteins contain nitrogen, an element essential to life. By weight, fats are the most concentrated sources of calories.

Inside your body's cells these three energy sources are broken down in a series of steps that release tiny increments of energy. Billions of these bursts of energy combine throughout your body to keep it running smoothly.

Carbohydrates : Simple and Complex

There are two types of carbohydrates: simple and complex. Simple carbohydrates are composed of relatively few building blocks (for example, glucose molecules) and are therefore broken down quickly and easily. Table sugar, honey, candy, jams and jellies, cakes and pastries are all examples of sources of simple carbohydrates. Usually a person's body releases enough insulin to clear the sugar from these simple carbohydrates out of the blood and move it into the cells, where it can be used for energy. In a diabetic, however, either there is not enough insulin to get the job done or the insulin is ineffective. The simple carbohydrates break down and flood into the bloodstream. That is why your physician will recommend that you limit simple carbohydrates if you have diabetes.

Complex carbohydrates present another story. These are much larger than the simple carbohydrates because they contain many building blocks. Complex carbohydrates are broken down slowly in the intestinal tract, and, as a result, even with decreased insulin, blood sugar rises much more slowly after you have eaten these foods. Starch found in pasta, bread, cereals, and vegetables, are examples of complex carbohydrates. Because these carbohydrates are broken down into their individual glucose units more slowly than simple carbohydrates, they do not affect the diabetic in the same way.

Recently many doctors have recommended that carbohydrates, especially the complex types, should make up 50 percent or more of the diabetic's total daily calories. In the past the percentage of carbohydrates in the diabetic's diet was considerably lower, the difference being made up by a higher percentage of fat in the diet. Now there is evidence that diets lower in total fat but with a greater proportion of polyunsaturated fat are helpful in preventing some forms of vascular disease. These facts, together with the knowledge that carbohydrates are not the risk or danger they were once thought to be, have greatly changed diets for people who have diabetes.

Insulin's Role in Controlling the Fuel Lines

Insulin acts to store the three energy-yielding components of your diet: carbohydrates, fat, protein. Further, it also helps prevent them from being broken down. Normally after a meal most of the carbohydrates derived from the food are stored in the liver with the assistance of insulin. Then between meals the liver produces glucose to prevent the blood sugar level from dropping too low. A major function of insulin is to prevent the liver from producing too much glucose.

This maintenance of your blood sugar level is vital to your brain, which must have glucose. If your brain does not get enough glucose, its function becomes impaired. On the other hand, if the blood sugar level rises too high due to a lack of insulin, the body's fat stores may begin to break down, flooding the bloodstream with acidic ketone bodies (the broken-down products from fat). A high level of these ketone bodies can cause a diabetic to become very ill. That is why it is important to maintain a fairly regular level of sugar in your blood because a high or low extreme can cause serious short- or long-term effects.

How does Weight Control Improve Insulin Action?

People who are overweight have fewer insulin receptor sites on the walls of their cells. Insulin receptor sites act as doors into the cells through which glucose can travel when insulin is attached to them. If there are fewer sites, more insulin is required to keep these doors open for the glucose. This increased need causes the insulin-producing cells in the pancreas to work much harder but less effectively, and their output of insulin may actually decrease. Then an even greater need for insulin arises, and there is a deficiency of it. While your cells may have extra glucose available, it can't be utilized. When you reduce your weight, however, you increase the number of receptor sites exposed on the cell walls. With more of these sites the need for insulin decreases and the cells in the pancreas are under less stress to produce, so they may recover some of their function and begin releasing more insulin. According to the American Diabetes Association this revitalization of the glucose-controlling mechanism can greatly reduce the severity of diabetes.

Calories, Diet, and Weight Control

Your physician and nutritionist will outline a diet plan to make the most efficient use of the food you eat. They will help you understand the relative nutritive and caloric values of various foods.

The calorie is a unit used to describe the energy content of food. One pound (about 454 grams) of body fat is equated with approximately 3,500 calories. Over the course of a week, if you adjust your diet so you eat 500 fewer calories each day, by the end

Optimum Weight* Chart
(Related to Height for Adults)

	Women				Men		
	Height		*Weight/kgs.*		*Height*		*Weight/kgs*
Ft	Ins	Cms	Range	Ft	Ins	Cms	Range
4	10	147.3	43.5-48.5				
4	11	149.9	44.5-49.9				
5	0	152.4	45.8-51.3	5	0	152.4	50.0-55.0
5	1	154.9	47.2-52.6	5	1	154.9	52.2-57.7
5	2	157.5	48.5-54.0	5	2	157.5	53.5-58.5
5	3	160.0	49.9-55.3	5	3	160.0	54.9-60.3
5	4	162.6	57.3-57.2	5	4	162.6	56.2-61.7
5	5	165.1	52.6-59.0	5	5	165.1	57.6-63.0
5	6	167.6	54.4-61.2	5	6	167.6	59.0-64.9
5	7	170.2	56.2-63.0	5	7	170.2	60.8-66.7
5	8	172.7	58.1-64.9	5	8	172.7	62.6-68.9
				5	9	175.3	64.4-70.8
				5	10	177.8	66.2-72.6
				5	11	180.3	68.0-74.8
				6	0	182.9	69.9-77.1

* For without clothes and shoes, subtract, 2.7. kg for women and 4.5 kg for men.

Source: *You Can Prevent Heart Attack* by Dr. O.P. Jaggi, published by Orient Paperbacks.

of the week, all other things being equal, you may have lost a pound with some variations, depending upon your size and metabolism. On the other hand, eating an extra 500 calories each day over the course of a week can slip an extra pound around your waist. (A large piece of apple pie is about 500 calories!)

How do the basic building blocks rate in terms of calories? Carbohydrates and proteins each have about four calories per gram. Fat is much higher at nine calories per gram.

Your physician may arrive at your ideal weight and your daily calorie allowance in several ways. A rough estimate sets the number of calories per day for maintenance of weight at 15 calories per pound of body weight. If you need to lose weight, you may be allotted only 10 calories per day per pound of body weight. Depending on several factors, such as the amount you exercise, your body build, and your age, these estimates might be slightly different.

Fiber Consumption and Diabetes

Your physician will explain the importance of including appropriate amounts of fiber in your new diet. Dietary fibers are constituents of plants that are not absorbed or metabolized by your small intestine and therefore reach your large intestine relatively unchanged. Dietary fiber is essential for normal function of your digestive tract. Fiber helps to retain water in your intestine, adds bulk to stools, softens them, and regulates the time it takes for food waste to move through the body. The addition of fiber to your meal in the form of wheat bran or whole grain foods, for example, slows the movement of food through your system and decreases the after-meal blood glucose levels and may lower the cholesterol level in your bloodstream.

What is a high-fiber diet? A typical high-fiber diet may contain two to three times as much fiber as a normal diet. Whole grains, fresh fruits, and fresh vegetables are all good sources of dietary fiber, especially the legumes, such as beans, lentils, and peas.

Scientists have data suggesting that fiber does more than reduce the after-meal blood glucose level. It has been found to improve the ability of the cells to receive and utilize insulin. Particularly in Type II (adult-onset) diabetes, reduction of the insulin requirement has occurred in patients even at their ideal weight. This may indicate that in the future this dietary approach to reducing insulin requirements in a large part of the adult-onset diabetic population will be even more important. An additional advantage may be the reduction of blood fat. Some researchers have even suggested that fiber in the diet reduces the chances of cancer of the gastrointestinal tract and other gastrointestinal disorders.

Table 4
Foods Containing Fiber Appropriate
for a Diabetic's Diet*

Food Item	Size of Serving	Fiber (grams)
Kidney beans, cooked	½ cup	1.4
Lima beans, cooked	½ cup	1.6
40% bran flakes	½ cup	1.1
Whole wheat bread	1 slice	.3
Cornflakes	¾ cup	1.7
Graham crackers	2-2½"	1.5
Lentils	½ cup	1.2
Peas	½ cup	1.5
Potatoes, cooked/mashed	½ cup	.4–.6
Broccoli	½ cup	1.2
Brussel sprouts	3-4	1.2
Carrots	½ cup	.6–.8
Eggplant	½ cup	.9
Parsnips, cooked	½ cup	2.2
Pea pods, Chinese	½ cup	1.4
Sauerkraut	½ cup	.8
Spinach	½ cup	.5
Tomato, fresh, with skin	1 small	.6

*Source : Adapted from recommendations of the American Diabetic Association.**

Diet for Insulin-Dependent Diabetics

Diet in therapy figures differently for insulin- and non-insulin-dependent diabetics. If you have insulin-dependent diabetes, your diet will require special attention. The timing of your meals is

** (See also Page 74)

very important. Insulin is taken to handle a predetermined diet, and that is why you must eat your meals on schedule and adhere to your doctor's prescribed diet. Depending on how much insulin you are taking and when, you may need to include snacks in your diet in the midmorning, the afternoon, and usually before bedtime. If you exercise, you will burn more calories than usual, and when you take your usual amount of insulin it will be necessary to balance this with extra calories. At times a reduced insulin intake will be recommended for extreme exercise you've planned, such as marathon running or long bicycle rides.

In insulin-dependent diabetics missed calories can lead to hypoglycemia, the condition in which the insulin in your system allows too much sugar to pass from your blood into your cells, thereby decreasing your blood sugar. Too many calories, on the other hand, means that your blood sugar will go up too much, and because the level of insulin remains constant, your blood sugar will remain too high.

Diet for Non-Insulin-Dependent Diabetics

If you do not take insulin, your prescribed diet may be geared primarily toward one goal, that of weight reduction. Although your body is still producing insulin, your problem may be that it isn't using the insulin very effectively. With reduced weight your insulin supply should remain sufficient, and your body is more likely to use it more effectively.

According to the American Diabetes Association and the American Dietetic Association, once non-insulin-dependent diabetics have lost enough to reach their ideal weight by cutting down on calories, most of them produce enough insulin to keep their blood sugar level normal. If you are like the majority of those in the non-insulin-dependent group, your chances of benefiting from weight control are excellent.

Exchange Lists and Meal Planning

Your doctor may put you on a 1,500-calorie-per-day diet, for example, from which 30 percent of the food you will eat is made up of fat, 15 percent protein, and 55 percent carbohydrates. What will you eat? How much of each food? Once such control was very confusing. But in 1950 exchange lists were developed, and for the first time diabetic diets became standardized. Before this system was introduced diabetics had to weigh their food carefully on a scale.

The American Dietetic Association, the American Diabetes Association, and the National Institutes of Health produce a publication called *Exchange Lists for Meal Planning*. This publication provides information about food composition and allows the diabetic to choose foods from various exchange lists (see Chapter 12 for addresses of these organizations). The booklet divides the diabetic's diet into six major exchange lists. Exchange lists afford you much more latitude in your diet. Foods in any one group can be substituted for or exchanged with other foods in the same group. Within each group an exchange is about equal in calories and amounts of carbohydrates, proteins, and fats; each exchange contains similar vitamins and minerals.

According to the American Diabetes Association and the American Dietetic Association, "No one exchange group can supply all the nutrients needed for a well-balanced diet. It takes all six of them working together as a team to supply your nutritional needs for good health."

The six exchanges are:

- *Milk exchanges:* Various types of milk and yogurt.
- *Vegetable exchanges:* When used raw, some vegetables may be used freely. Such free vegetables include lettuce, radishes, parsley, dill pickles, and cucumbers. Starchy vegetables are counted in the bread exchange list.
- *Fruit exchanges:* Fruits; many of them are high in vitamin A or C and potassium. (Remember that fruits are high in simple sugars and require careful measurement.)
- *Bread exchanges:* Bread, cereal, and starchy vegetables such as corn, potatoes, and peas.
- *Meat exchanges:* These are divided into three subcategories: lean meat, medium-fat meat, and high-fat meat. (These may

vary by as much as 40 calories per ounce, depending on the group.) Included in the meat exchanges are meats, fish, poultry, and other protein-rich foods, such as cheese, beans, and peas. *Fat exchanges:* Both vegetable and animal fats. (Most vegetable fats are polyunsaturated, whereas animal fats are high in saturated fats.)

You will learn to limit certain foods, particularly those high in carbohydrates (see list below).

Foods to Use in a Limited way

Sugar
Candy
Soft drinks
Some beverages

Foods That Can Be Used in an Unlimited Way

Calorie-free soft drinks	Boiled meat without fat
Decaffeinated coffee	Seasoning such as lemon
Tea (somewhat limited)	and lime, garlic, paprika,
	cinnamon, vinegar, mint,
	herbs

Foods high in simple carbohydrates, such as sugar, candy, and soft drinks, may be used in minimal ways if you calculate them into your diet plan. For example, although catsup may include sugar, the amount you use may be insignificant and may not affect your overall sugar intake. Sugar-coated pills, regular chewing gum, and cough medicine contribute small amounts of glucose (sugar) and may be used carefully for the short-term with your physician's permission. They may be better than using a sugar substitute, which may cost you more money and may cause undesirable side effects. When you have questions about use of any foods that are not on your list of approved foods, check with your health care team. Also, it is important to read labels and be aware of not only the presence but also the amounts of sugar and calories.

In planning your menus with your health care team, exchange lists prepared by the American Diabetes Association and other organizations may be helpful to you. Suggestions for obtaining these lists are included in the reading list in Chapter 12.

Controlling Your Diabetes: Change Your Eating Habits

Losing weight may be enough to stabilize your diabetes. It can work, if you do it carefully and thoughtfully, under your physician's supervision.

In an effort to lose weight, many people conduct a never-ending search for the "perfect" diet, the one that *really* works. They regain the weight between diets because they are really never quitting their old eating habits. In the past few years a multitude of new diets have been developed. If any of these new fad diets were so effective in reducing weight, why would so many more continue to appear? Most medical authorities agree that the best diet for weight loss in a person who has diabetes is a properly calculated and distributed one. You must be aware of your nutritional intake. You can save your health dollar and select your sources of diet information wisely. To reduce your weight and keep it down you need more than a miracle diet. You need an understanding of the basics of nutrition. And if you ask yourself why you eat, you may find some revelations. Do you eat when you have problems? Do you eat when you're angry, happy, lonely, or as a reward? Why do you overeat?

There have been many health fads in which claims were made that diet alone can be used to treat diabetes without insulin injections. While it is true that there are conditions in which calorie control and high fiber are highly beneficial to the person with diabetes, such a diet must be followed only under the supervision of a diabetes-oriented health care team.

Dieting Tips

Losing weight can be easy: take in fewer calories. On paper,

anyway, this seems simple. Many people's ha
ingrained; they may seem impossible to cł
change your eating habits, especially when d
trolling your disease.

Eat regular meals and avoid deviating
eating schedule. Do not leave food out wł___ ___ ___ see it
between meals. If you do, you'll be more than likely to eat it.
Don't watch TV while you eat. Try to keep eating and social
activities separate.

When you shop for food, keep several things in mind. Never
shop when you're hungry. Instead, shop from a prepared shopping list and try to stick to it. Read labels. The fact that a label
says a product is "dietetic" does not mean you can eat unlimited
quantities of it. Learn to spot sugar on labels. It may be listed
several times under several names. Buy unprocessed foods that
you can prepare at home. You have more control over what goes
into your meals this way.

Table 5
How to Spot Sugar on Food Labels

Name	Meaning
Brown Sugar	Sucrose crystals covered with a film of syrup.
Confectioner's Sugar	Powdered sucrose.
Corn Sugar	Sugar made from cornstarch.
Dextrin	Glucose molecules that may affect body in the same way as glucose.
Dextrose	Another name for glucose; contains calories.
Dulcitol	A sugar made from alcohol.
Fructose	A naturally occurring sugar found in fruit and honey. Although the sweetness of fructose varies, it can be twice as sweet as sucrose. Contains calories.
Glucose	A naturally occurring simple sugar, about half as sweet as table sugar. Dextrose is the commercial name for glucose and may be seen on food labels. Glucose and dextrose contain calories.

How to Spot Sugar on Food Labels (cont.)

Name	Meaning
Glucose Syrups	These are liquid sweeteners containing a mixture of glucose, maltose, and other glucose molecules. Corn syrup solids are the crystallized form of corn syrup. Glucose syrups have calories.
Granulated Sugar	Sucrose. Caloric.
Honey	Syrup made largely from fructose.
Invert Sugar	A combination of sugars from fruits.
Lactose	The sugar found in milk.
Maltose	The sugar formed by the breakdown of starch.
Mannitol	A sugar alcohol broken down by the body in the same way as other sugars but absorbed more slowly.
Sorbitol	A sugar alcohol produced from glucose and invert sugar but absorbed more slowly than table sugar.
Sorghum	A syrup made from sorghum grain.
Sucrose	Another name for table sugar. Caloric.

Reduce the Risk of Cardiovascular Disease Through Diet

Diabetes, obesity, high blood pressure, a high-cholesterol level, cigarette smoking, lack of exercise, and emotional stress are all risk factors for coronary artery and other vascular diseases. Diabetes increases your risk of getting these diseases, particularly if it is combined with any other risk factors. If you have diabetes, you should be very careful to avoid the other risk factors of coronary artery disease. You can do this by being aware that fat and salt intake are two common culprits in cardiovascular disease. Too much salt in most people's diets may cause their blood pressure to rise. This high blood pressure, or hypertension, puts extra strain on the heart and blood vessels. Hypertension can also aggravate atherosclerosis, a condition marked by hardened and clogged arteries. In turn, as atherosclerosis becomes more severe, so does hypertension.

Fat and cholesterol consumption has been linked by many researchers to atherosclerosis. Persons whose cholesterol level is too high are more likely to develop hardened and clogged arteries. A group of fats called *saturated fats* are commonly believed to be the fats at fault. Saturated fats are normally derived from animal products and are usually solid at room temperature. Examples are butter and bacon. Fats obtained from vegetable products are known as *unsaturated fats*; they are usually liquid at room temperature. These unsaturated fats are generally not considered any menace to health when eaten in moderation.

Blood Cholesterol Value Chart*

Normal *(mg. per 100 ml* *of Blood)*	180-250 mg
High *(mg. per 100 ml* *of Blood)*	250 mg. and above

*Source : WHO

Watch What You Eat

At first you may consider following the diet your doctor has prescribed somewhat of a nuisance because it requires planning your own meals in addition to meals for the rest of your family. However, you will probably be like most diabetics, who become enthusiastic about what they eat because good eating habits are good living habits and share their diets with their families as good dietary habits.

Diet is important to everyone, diabetics as well as nondiabetics. Yours is a personal diet, planned to help you lead a happier, healthier life.

Diabetes Meal Planner

Diet constitutes an essential part of treatment of diabetes mellitus. The restriction in diet is generally misinterpreted as abstenance from all rich and tasty meals. In fact diabetics need more nourishing and better balanced diet than normal people because of certain limitations in their metabolism. In an attempt to normalize blood sugar essential nutrients required for normal growth and development should not be sacrificed.

For a successful management patients must understand their daily food requirements, nutritive values of food items and how to select foods to avoid monotony and embarrassing social situations. Special adjustments are required in case of treatment with Insulin, specially short acting Insulin, or acute illnesses like infections, diarrhoea and vomiting or for social, religious occasions like fasts, festivals and get-togethers.

The doctors and dieticians can help you to ascertain your individual requirements according to your age, weight, sex, physical activities and suggest you the ideal meal pattern. But your own knowledge of food values will go a long way in stabilizing your diabetes and enjoying life inspite of the disease.

Normally a Diabetic Requires

- 25 to 30 Kilocalories (Kcal) per Kg body weight
- 1 to 1.5g Proteins per Kg body weight
- 30 to 50g Fat (preferably 30g unsaturated)
- 200 to 300g Carbohydrates(CHO), mainly starch not sugar.
- Fibres : Fruits, vegetables and cereals contain more fibre.
- Vitamins and minerals

Standard 1500 Kcal diet of Indian meal pattern along with its calculations of Calories and nutrients (Protein, Fat and Carbohydrate) is presented for your guidance. The food exchange lists have been prepared for selecting alternatives to provide variety and to break the monotony of meal pattern. The exchanges can be used for increasing or decreasing the Calorie or Nutrient allowances from the standard 1500 Kcal diet, if so, advised by your doctor.*

---

* Source : Diabetic Self-Care Foundation, India.

Doctor! What Should Be My Diet?

Avoid

- Sugar in any form—sweets, ice-cream, kulfi, chocolates, candy etc.
- Vegetables with high starch content like potatoes, colocasia *(arbi)*, sweet potatoes, yam etc.
- Refined cereal products like semolina *(suji)*, white flour *(maida)*, wheat-flour *without* bran and rice (unless you are a rice eater).
- Milk and milk products with cream or fat, such as *khoya*, curd, yoghurt, cheese (paneer), made out of full or whole cream milk etc.
- Ghee and butter, fried preparation like puri, parantha, samosa, pokora etc.
- Fruits with high sugar or starch content like banana, sapota *(chiku)*, grapes, lichees, mango etc.
- Egg-yolk, keema, ham, sausages, organ meat like liver, kidney, brain etc.
- Wines and beer.

Instead

- Use artificial sweeteners.
- Take green vegetables, rich in fibre like bittergourd, bottlegourd, lettuce leaves, leeks, french beans, brinjals, ladies fingers, cabbage, cauliflower, carrot, soyabeans, drumsticks etc; take vegetables with moderate calories like peas, beet root, jack fruit *(kathal)*. onions etc. in smaller quantity.
- Take wheat flour *with* bran, rice after eliminating its *starch water*.
- Take skimmed milk and products like curd, yoghurt, cheese etc. made out of skimmed milk.
- Use oil as cooking medium; baked, tandoori or grilled preparations should be preferred.
- Take orange, watermelon, sweet lemon, apple etc.
- Take white of egg, white meat like fish, chicken lamb.
- Take spirits like whisky, brandy in moderation.

Standard 1500 K Cal Indian Diet

Cantaining Carbohydrates 215 g, Proteins 70 g, Fat 40 g with Daily Allowance
Milk 500 ml, Oil 15 g

	Kcal	CHO	Protein	Fat
Bed Tea No Sugar				
Breakfast				
Porridge 20 g*	68	13.8	2.4	0.3
or Slice (1) 30g	70	15.0	2.4	0.3
Egg 1	78	—	6.0	6.0
Or Paneer 30 g	79	0.3	5.5	6.2
or Cheese 25 g	87	1.6	6.0	6.2
Slice 1	70	15.0	2.4	0.3
or Chapati 20 g	68	13.8	2.4	0.3
or Idli 1/3 Rice	69	13.0	2.9	0.2
Milk 1 Cup	114	7.7	5.5	7.0
Mid-Morning				
Tea/Coffee				
Fruits/Biscuits	70	12.0	1.0	3.0
Lunch				
Salad 125 g	35	6.0	3.0	—
Mixed veg 100 g	35	7.0	2.0	—
Dal 30 g	100	170	6.7	0.6

or Paneer 35 g	93	0.4	6.4	7.3
or Mutton 50 g	97	—	9.3	6.7
or Chicken 70 g	105	—	17.0	4.0
or Fish 100 g	91	—	20.0	—
Chapati 2	*136*	*27.6*	*4.8*	*0.6*
Curd 130 ml	*80*	*5.3*	*3.8*	*4.8*
Tea Tea				
Fruits/Biscuits	*70*	*16.0*	*1.0*	*—*
or Glucose	68	10.8	1.0	2.2
or Salted	80	8.2	1.0	4.4
Dinner				
Soup	*10*	*2.5*	*—*	*—*
Salad 125 g	*35*	*6.0*	*3.0*	*—*
(Mixed) 100 g	*35*	*7.0*	*2.0*	*—*
Dal 30 g	*100*	*17.0*	*67*	*0.6*
Curd 120 ml	*80*	*5.3*	*3.8*	*4.8*
Chapati 2	*136*	*27.6*	*48*	*0.6*
Milk (Bed Time)	*114*	*7.7*	*5.5*	*7.0*

* Items in italics have high carbohydrate content.

Protein Exchange Equivalent of One Egg
(6.4 g Protein)

Food	Quantity (edible portion) gram	Kilo Calorie	Protein gram
Egg large	45	78	6.4
Cow's Milk	200ml	135	6.4
Buffalo's Milk *	*150ml*	*175*	*6.4*
Homogenised Milk	150ml	100	6.4
Skimmed Milk	250ml	72	6.4
Paneer(cow's milk)	*35*	*93*	*6.4*
Paneer(buffalo's milk)	*50*	*146*	*6.7*
Cheese	*25*	*87*	*6.0*
Chicken fryer, flesh	25	27	6.4
Chicken broiler, flesh	25	38	6.4
Liver (goat)	30	32	6.0
Kidney	40	42	6.8
Brain	*65*	*81*	*6.5*
Mutton (muscle)	35	78	6.5
Pork lean muscle	30	34	5.6

Sausages	60	270	*6.6*
Bacon fried	*25*	*151*	*6.2*
Ham	*25*	*100*	*6.0*
Fish (without skin & bone)	35	31	6.4
Crab muscles (cooked 40 gm)	70	41	6.2
Prawns	35	31	6.7
Soyabean	15	65	6.4
Average dal	30	104	6.4
Peanut butter	*30*	*93*	*6.4*
Channa roasted	30	110	6.4
Rajmah	30	104	6.8
Peas green (fresh)	90	84	6.5

Note : Calories to be adjusted by including/excluding equal quantity of carbohydrate.
* Foods in italics have higher fat content hence to be avoided/adjusted.

Carbohydrate Exchange Equivalent of One Chappati (20 g Atta)

Food	Quantity (edible portion) gram	Kilo Calorie	Carbohydrates gram
Cereals & Products			
Atta (thin, small saucer size chapati)	20	68	13.9
Rice raw milled (1 cup)*	20	68	15.6
Bread white (1 slice large loaf)	28.5	70	14.8
Bread brown (1 slice)	28.5	70	13.9
Biscuits salted (4)	12	65	6.6
Biscuits sweet (2 glucose or 4 crackjack)	15	68	10.8
Oats porridge (2/3 cup)	20	65	12.6
Maize (½ roti) or cornflakes 2/3 cup	20	68	13.2
Popcorn (1½ cups)	15	67	9.0
Kootu (1 small roti)	20	65	13.0
Water chestnut flour	20	65	13.8
Jowar	20	68	14.5
Rice flakes (pale)	20	68	15.5
Rice puffed (murmure)	20	65	14.7

Item			
Wheat dalia	20	68	*14.0*
Wheat suji	20	68	*14.2*
Sponge cake plain (1¼" section of 8" cake)	25	73	13.5
Dals & Beans			
Dal (average)	20	68	11.6
Rajmah	20	68	12.1
Chana kabuli or Bengal gram	20	68	12.2
Baked beans (in tomato suce ½ cup)	60	73	13.8
Vegetable			
Carrots	140	70	14.8
Arbi/Potato	70	70	*15.4*
Water chestnut	60	69	*14.0*
Average salad vegetable	250	70	10.0
Leafy vegetable	150	66	10.5
Other vegetable (summer)	250	70	10.5
Other vegetable (winter)	200	72	11.0
Beetroot	160	70	14.1
Lotus root	130	70	14.7
Onion	150	75	16.6
Radish (2 large)	400	60	13.6

* Items in italics have high carbohydrate content.

Food	Quantity (edible portion.) gram	Kilo Calorie	Carbohydrates gram
Sweet potato	*60*	*68*	*16.9*
Yam	*85*	*68*	*15.6*
Fruits			
Apple (1 medium peeled)	120	72	16.0
Banana (½ large or 1 small)	*60*	*65*	*16.3*
Peach (2 small or 1 large)	150	75	15.7
Pear (2 small or 1 large)	125	65	14.9
Plums (2 medium size)	125	65	13.9
Papaya (¼ medium sized fruit)	225	72	16.2
Orange 2 medium sized)	150	72	16.4
Mussamies (1½ medium size)	150	63	14.0
Malta	200	72	15.6
Grapes palegreen (1 small bunch)	100	71	16.5
Water melon 3" slice	450	72	14.8
Musk melon (½ medium size fruit)	400	68	14.0
Lichi (5-6 lichis)	125	73	17.0
Guava 1 medium	125	64	14.0

* Items in italics have high carbohydrate content.

Fat Exchange
(Approx 15 mg fat portion) (1 Table Spoon ghee)

Food	Quantity edible portion) gram	Kilo Calorie	Protein gram
Butter	20	140	15.0
Cream (heavy, whipping)	40	135	15.8
Mayonnaise	20	138	15.0
Ghee (cow's or buffalo's milk)	15	135	15.0
Ghee vanaspati (Hydrogenated)	15	135	15.0
Cooking oil; mustard oil, palm oil, gingely ground nut; cotton seed oil, coconut oil, lineseed oil, refined oils, eg. Ruby oil, Dalda Refined, Marvo, Postman, Saffola, Safflower Oil sun flower oil etc.	15	135	15.0

Fibre Content of Foods
(Per 100 gms. edible portion)

Food	Fibre gram
Pulses and Legumes	
Green gram (Mung)	4.1
Green gram dal (Mung dal)	0.8
Black gram (Urd dal)	0.9
Bengal gram dal (Channa dal)	1.2
Lentil (Masur dal)	0.7
Red Gram (Tur dal)	1.5
Soyabeans	3.7
Vegetables	
Cabbage	1
Cauliflower	1.2
Carrots	1.2
Coriander leaves	1.2
Cucumber	0.4
Brinjals	1.3
Bittergourd	0.8
Drumstick	5
Ladies Fingers (Bhindi)	1.2
Leeks	1.3
Lettuce leaves	0.5
Mint (Pudina)	2
Fenugreek leaves (Methi ka Sag)	1.1
French-beans	1.8
Beet root	1
Onions (small)	0.6
Onions (mature)	0.6
Peas Green (fresh)	4
Potatoes (Alu)	0.4
Sweet Potatoes	0.8
Radish (Muli)	0.8

Food	Fibre gram
Spinach (Palak)	0.6
Tomatoes (fresh)	0.8
Tomato juice	0.25
Fruits	
Apples	1.0
Apricots (fresh)	1
Bananas (ripe)	0.4
Cherries (red)	0.4
Currants (black)	1
Dates (fresh)	4
Figs	2.2
Grapes (green variety)	3
Guava (country)	5.2
Jack fruit	1
Lemon (Sour lime)	2
Lemon (sweet)	0.7
Lichees	0.5
Mango (ripe)	0.7
Malon (water)	0.2
Orange	0.3
Papaya (ripe)	0.8
Peaches	1.2
Pears	1.0
Pineapple	0.5
Plums (red)	0.4
Pomegranate	5.1
Raisin (Khishmish)	1.1
Seetaphal (Custard apple)	3.1
Sapota (Chiku)	2.6
Strawberries	1.1
Sugar-cane	3
Sugar-cane juice	3
Cereal and Cereal foods	
Bajra	1

Food	Fibre gram
Barley	4
Jowar	1.6
Oatmeal	3.5
Rice raw (milled)	0.2
Rice raw (unmilled)	0.6
Wheat flour (Whole Atta)	2
Wheat flour refined (Maida)	0.3
Bread (White)	0.2
Wheat gram	1.4

Nuts and Seeds

Food	Fibre gram
Almonds	2
Cashew-nuts	1
Coconut (dried)	7
Ground-nuts (rosted)	3
Pistachio nuts	2
Walnuts	3

Daily Allowance At A glance
Standard 1500 K Cal Diabetic Diet

Food	Qty in gram	Kilo Calorie (Kcal)	Protein gram	Fat gram	Carbyhydrate (CHO) gram
Cow's Milk	500	335	16.0	20.5	22.0
Egg (One)	45	78	6.0	6.0	—
Dal	60	200	13.5	1.2	35.0
Bread	60	140	4.8	0.6	30.0
Biscuits (Salto)	15	68	1.0	4.5	7.5
Atta (Salto)	80	272	8.0	2.0	56.0
Leafy Veg.	150	66	5.0	1.0	9.0
Salad Veg.	250	70	8.0	—	27.0
Veg.(Winter/Summer)	200	70	—	—	—
Fruit	100 to 150	70	—	—	15.7
Oil (cooking)	15	135	—	15.0	—
		1504	62.3	50.8	202.2

5

Exercise, Food and Insulin

Exercise, appropriate diet, a good mental attitude, and, if necessary, insulin or an antidiabetes agent are the fundamentals of diabetes control. In Chapter 4 we discussed diet; here we turn our attention to exercise and how this aspect of your treatment interacts with those of diet and medication.

Your doctor will discuss with you the importance of balancing these factors and recommend appropriate forms of exercise on a regular basis. Jogging in the park, walking, playing racquetball, bicycling, windsurfing, dancing, playing sandlot baseball—choose your favorite and help your physician design a routine that will be both helpful in controlling your diabetes and enjoyable.

What Can Exercise do for You?

Most important, exercise can help you control your weight; it also makes insulin more effective in lowering your blood glucose level and aiding the entry of glucose into the cells. It can also increase the efficiency of your lungs and heart, help reduce hypertension, help you handle stress by relieving physical tension, and reduce the cholesterol level in your bloodstream.

While exercise can be of great value to both insulin-dependent diabetics and non-insulin-dependent diabetics, there are some differences in the ways exercise affects each group of people.

Exercise and the Insulin-Dependent Diabetic

If you are an insulin-dependent diabetic, understanding how exercise affects your body can help you avoid hypoglycemia and hyperglycemia. Either can result from exercise if you do not plan your schedule carefully. If insulin-dependent, you will find that you must adhere more closely to your daily schedule than a non-insulin-dependent diabetic. Generally, just as you plan to eat your meals and take your insulin at the same time each day, you will also want to schedule your exercise routine with regularity.

Exercise increases your muscles' demands for glucose because working muscles use more energy than relaxed muscles. This energy is derived from the glucose circulating in your bloodstream. In this way exercise helps lower your blood sugar level.

If you take insulin injections, the kind of exercise you do may influence your insulin injection site because exercise can increase the rate of absorption of insulin by your body from the injection site. Researchers have found that when insulin is injected into an exercising limb, such as your leg, as you are walking or running it is absorbed faster. This is not desirable because the fast absorption may actually cause the injected insulin to act too quickly on your system. Therefore, after planning your exercise program, your physician will suggest injection sites in parts of your body not being exercised.

In many cases an increased sensitivity to insulin is beneficial, as it may decrease the amount of insulin you have to take. If you are taking insulin, however, you should carefully balance the insulin with the food you eat and the amount of exercise you get. When you exercise you will learn to adjust either your insulin injections or the amount you eat. If you are overweight, however, your doctor may recommend that you lower your insulin injections rather than increase your food consumption. This way you will burn more calories and eat no extra food, so you should be able to reduce your weight. Because the kind and duration of your exercise cannot always be anticipated, it may be easier to increase your food intake before exercising.

When is the best time to exercise? Usually the best time is 15 minutes to two hours after a meal, since your blood sugar is higher then than at any other time. If you think you need extra 'food, try to eat it about 15 minutes before you exercise. If you exercise vigorously for extended periods of time, you may require some extra food about every half hour. Occasionally after you finish exercising you may still notice signs of hypoglycemia; at those times you may also require food. Especially during all-day activities, such as hiking or a long bicycle ride, you will want to be well prepared with extra food. You can easily carry a concentrated form of high-energy snacks. Sugar cubes, hard candies, and orange juice are examples of foods that can raise blood sugar that has been reduced too much by exercise. If you do become hypoglycemic, eat extra food until your symptoms subside or your blood sugar returns to normal. After your blood sugar has returned to normal, if it is not near mealtime, it may be advisable to eat some complex carbohydrates (such as bread, cereal, or other starchy food) to keep your blood glucose level stabilized.

In determining a time for exercise, consider when the action of your insulin peaks. Insulin may peak anywhere from about 2 to 12 hours after the injection, depending on the kind you inject. Exercising at the time that your insulin peaks is not a good idea because the combination of exercise and high insulin level could reduce your blood sugar too much, causing hypoglycemia.

Patients on insulin pumps may need to reprogram their pumps for exercise. (See Chapter 11.)

Exercise for Uncontrolled Diabetics

If you are an insulin-dependent-diabetic, at times when your diabetes is out of control your physician will tell you that the presence of ketones in your urine is an indication that your body is not using glucose from your bloodstream appropriately. When you exercise, your blood glucose automatically rises in response to your body's call for more energy. Such a rise, coupled with your body's inability to use glucose, could lead to even greater hyperglycemia. But you may have ketones in your urine after doing exercise with low blood sugar because your body is burning fats to produce glucose to keep the blood sugar normal. When this occurs, extra food, *not* insulin, is necessary.

Exercise for Non-Insulin-Dependent Diabetics

If you are a non-insulin dependent diabetic and are overweight, your main goal will probably be to lose weight through exercise. According to the American Diabetes Association, "Losing weight usually results in a dramatic reversal of diabetes and prevents many serious complications of diabetes." The following table shows approximately how many calories are used up during various types of exercise.

Table 6
How Calories and Activities Relate*

Activity	Calories Expended Per Hour
Light	**50–199**
Lying down or sleeping	80
Sitting	100
Driving a car	120
Standing	140
Housework	180
Moderate	**200–299**
Walking (4.25 Kms)	210
Bicycling (8.25 Kms)	210
Gardening	220
Canoeing (4.25 Kms)	230
Golf	250
Lawn mowing (power mower)	250
Lawn mowing (hand mower)	270
Bowling	270
Marked	**300–399**
Fencing	300
Rowing (4.25 Kms)	300
Swimming (400 mtrs)	300
Walking (6 Kms)	300
Badminton	350
Horseback riding (trotting)	350
Square-dancing	350
Volleyball	350
Roller-skating	350
Table tennis	360

* These calorie expenditures are approximations.

How Calories and Activities Relate (cont.)

Activity	Calories Expended Per Hour
Vigorous	**>400**
Ice-skating (16 Kms)	400
Wood chopping or sawing	400
Tennis	420
Hill climbing (30.5 mtrs)	480
Skiing (16 Kms)	490
Squash	600
Handball	600
Bicycling (21 Kms)	660
Running (16 Kms)	900

Scientists say that the cells of obese people may have only half as many insulin receptors as those of slender people. With fewer insulin receptors their cells are not able to respond adequately to the amount of insulin in their system, and the blood sugar rises. Losing weight has been known to increase the number of these receptors. Losing weight removes the stress that obesity imposes on the beta cells in the pancreas (the cells that make insulin) because with an increased number of receptor sites less insulin is needed and less is produced. If you are overweight, the longer you remain overweight, the more strain these cells are under, until eventually they may actually shut down completely. Even if you don't lose weight, exercise can increase the sensitivity of your insulin receptors to insulin, which in turn can reduce the stress placed on the beta cells.

Exercise, Hypertension and Diabetes

Exercise can also lower your blood pressure. This is important because high blood pressure, or hypertension, is one of several contributing factors leading to coronary artery disease. Other contributing factors are cigarette smoking, obesity, high blood cholesterol level, stress, and diabetes. Any one of these factors alone increases a person's chances of coronary artery disease, but any combination of two or more greatly increases the chances. Therefore, because you already have diabetes, you will want to do everything possible to avoid the other contributing factors for coronary artery disease.

Exercise, Cholesterol and Diabetes

Exercise and diet may help you lower an elevated blood cholesterol level. This is important because a high cholesterol level has been linked with atherosclerosis. Hardening of the arteries increases the likelihood or intensity of hypertension, and hypertension in turn can cause further atherosclerosis. If this cycle isn't already vicious enough, diabetes can increase the likelihood of atherosclerosis and hypertension or speed their development if they are already present.

Exercise may reduce the blood cholesterol level because exercise increases the amount of proteins in your bloodstream known as high-density lipoproteins (HDLs), which are responsible for removing cholesterol from your bloodstream.

Your Personal Exercise Program

Your physician and health care team will help you choose an exercise program that is best for you. They will tell you about two types of exercise, aerobic and anaerobic. Aerobic exercise is exercise that uses oxygen to help create energy for your muscles. This type of exercise increases the efficiency of your heart, muscles, lungs, and blood vessels. These conditioning effects, however, depend on exercising often enough, hard enough, and for long enough. Good examples of aerobic exercise are walking and bicycling, swimming, and running. Racquetball, paced calisthenics, and tennis are good examples of more active aerobic exercise.

Anaerobic exercise is exercise in which your muscles derive energy without the help of oxygen. Without oxygen muscles can achieve great bursts of energy that are not immediately dependent on available oxygen but will soon go into oxygen debt. Additionally, chemical by-products of the substances broken down for energy can pool up in your muscles and cause fatigue. While this type of exercise may stress the muscles used, it will not condition your cardiovascular system. A good example of anerobic exercise is running for a bus, when you exert yourself in an all-out effort and feel out of breath when you climb aboard. What happens is that you have used up oxygen at a faster rate than you took it in, resulting in oxygen debt. This is in contrast to regular jogging, an aerobic exercise, during which your use of oxygen does not exceed your intake.

You will probably want to concentrate on aerobic exercise to condition your cardiovascular system. In time aerobic exercise can decrease your resting and exercise heart rates, which means that your heart works less hard to do its job. To reach this point, however, you must exercise at least three times per week, or every other day. If you exercise less often than this, you will not actually be conditioning your body. In fact, the weekend athlete is more likely to strain a muscle or incur some injury than achieve any good effect. Also, if you have been regularly exercising aerobically and you suddenly decrease your exercise schedule to fewer than three times a week, you will lose whatever benefits you have gained. Exercise must be a regular activity to produce any benefit.

The next factor involved in aerobic conditioning is effort, how hard you push yourself. In order to achieve cardiovascular conditioning some physicians say you must perform at 70–85 percent of your maximum heart rate. There are two ways to find your maximum heart rate. One way is simply to push yourself to the limit and record your pulse until it goes no higher. If you are middle-aged, your doctor may suggest that you do just this, under supervision, of course, in an exercise stress test. In an exercise stress test you run on a treadmill or pedal a stationary bike until you attain your maximum heart rate. While you are doing this an electrocardiogram will show the tester how you are reacting to the stress. An easier way to obtain your approximate maximum heart rate is to subtract your age from 220. For example, if you are 40 years old, your maximum heart rate would be 220 – 40 = 180. If you exceed 85 percent of this maximal heart rate you may actually harm yourself, while if you exercise at much less than 70 percent of this maximal heart rate, the exercise is probably not effective in developing cardiovascular fitness.

How Much Exercise is Too Much?

In addition to regularity and intensity, the duration of your exercise is important. How long is long enough? Your physician will probably suggest that you do at least a half hour of continuous activity. During this time your pulse should be held to within 70–85 percent of maximum. You will be advised not to expect to be able to go out and reach this level of aerobic exercise immediately after you begin your exercise program. This is something that you will build up to gradually. Most people take from several weeks to several months to reach this level.

All exercise plans should include warm-up and cool-down periods. The entire exercise session should last about one hour. Plan to begin with 10–15 minutes of stretching, bending, and warming up. This will loosen up your muscles so they are not suddenly jolted when you begin your exercise. After exercising for about 30 minutes, cool down by gradually coming to rest or perhaps doing more stretching and bending.

If you have not exercised much in the past, you should begin your exercise program slowly. Walking is an excellent way to begin. It is easy and economical and can be done anytime, anywhere. Both walking and jogging have become popular forms of exercise because they can be done consistently and they easily fit into most people's schedules. If you are beginning an exercise program, exercises such as dancing, hiking, and team sports may not be the best way to begin. These activities may take more effort than you expect, and the efforts you expend are not as easily controlled as in walking or jogging.

Are any Exercises Off Limits?

While some physicians place no limitations on activities for diabetics whose diseases are under control, the American Diabetes Association advises against certain sports: "Although many athletic endeavors are open to diabetics, certain activities should definitely be avoided in order to prevent harm to yourself or others. Basically, these involve situations where a hypoglycemic reaction could lead to disaster. That's why scuba diving, parachuting, and mountain climbing are less desirable choices for people with diabetes and require much greater care while swimming, hiking, and most team sports are usually fine."

If you are interested in any of these activities, you will want to discuss their appropriateness for you with your own health care team. Your physician will advise you not to exercise if you are ill and to avoid exercising during extremes in weather or on smoggy days. You will be reminded to drink enough water to replace liquids lost through perspiration.

Enjoy!

Exercise, like diet and medication (if your doctor has prescribed any), is something that will provide benefits only if it becomes part of your lifestyle. So choose an exercise you enjoy. Perhaps you will want to encourage others in your family to run with you or join a tennis or softball game. Your exercise hobby can be a great source of pleasure. Regular exercise can improve your muscle tone, help control your weight, decrease tension, increase stamina, and make your world a happier place.

6

Pregnancy and Other Special Concerns of Women

You may be one of about 1½ million women in their childbearing years who have diabetes. You can deliver healthy, normal babies even though you are diabetic. With careful medical supervision and control of your disease your chances of fertility and successful delivery are nearly as good as those of nondiabetic women.

Because you are diabetic, you will face more stresses during pregnancy than nondiabetic women. You will also contend with the same uncertainties shared by all expectant mothers. You will face some occasional discomfort, such as "morning sickness," an increased chance of having bladder infections and varicose veins, and weight gain. You will be aware that your physical appearance is changing and that you are treated in special ways by family members. At times you may feel irritable and depressed for no apparent reason. You may notice that interest in affection and sex may increase or decrease for you and your spouse. Still, despite these concerns, your pregnancy will be a time of happy anticipation and shared expectations with your husband and family.

Better management of diabetes as well as pregnancy have improved the outlook for childbearing by the diabetic woman over the past 25 years. Because, however, the statistical chances for a diabetic woman to deliver an infant with a birth defect are greater than for nondiabetic women, it is essential that your pregnancy be diagnosed early and that you have regular blood tests and examinations to monitor blood factors important to control of your diabetes and to your baby's growth and development.

Special Care During Pregnancy

While all 40 weeks of your pregnancy are important to your baby's growth and development, the first 12 weeks are the most critical time for normal fetal organ development. Keeping control of your diabetes can prevent damage to your baby at that time. During the first trimester you will also store nutrients, largely in the form of fat, which the fetus will use later on. Having your diabetes well under control can prevent problems such as excess insulin production in the baby, which in turn can cause the baby to have low blood sugar after birth or possibly genetic changes that may contribute to a potential for developing diabetes.

A known diabetic should try to avoid entering into pregnancy without a period of tight control before the pregnancy. If your diabetes was under control before pregnancy, you will probably be able to control it easily during your pregnancy and have few new difficulties. If it was not under control prior to pregnancy, however, you may find that you have an even higher sugar level. Also, you may find that you need a reduction in insulin, if you are an insulin-dependent diabetic, and that you will require a diet adjustment. (As a precaution, it will be helpful to teach someone else in your household how to give you glucagon injections in case you have any severe reactions and cannot take carbohydrates by mouth.)

First Trimester

Your dietary goal during the first trimester should be to eat enough food for you and your baby but to avoid high blood sugar and insulin reactions. You probably will be advised by your physician to follow a diet that is higher in calories and particularly in protein because protein is essential to developing healthy tissues in your baby. You will be advised not to lose weight during pregnancy, even if you are overweight, because the baby may not receive enough required nutrients if you go on a reducing diet. Your physician will probably recommend a diet consisting of sufficient calories per day and supplemental calcium, vitamins, and protein. Depending on your height and body build, you should expect a weight gain of 20–25 pounds to assure good health for you and your baby. The diet should be adequate to avoid ketones in the urine.

Testing will be an important part of your personal care routine during pregnancy. You may be advised to change your method of testing at this time. Also, you may be a patient of a medical center that advises women to use home blood testing with strips or meters. Urine testing for sugar and ketones may be recommended. (You will learn more about self-testing in Chapter 8.)

While you are pregnant you may notice more glucose than usual in your urine. Your physician will explain that this will occur even if your blood sugar is not higher than before. This may not indicate that your diabetes is getting out of control. During pregnancy, you should also test for ketones. There is more danger of going into a diabetic coma (ketoacidosis) with a high sugar reading during pregnancy than at other times, and ketones during pregnancy may indicate difficulties for mother and baby.

During pregnancy your eyes and kidneys should also be evaluated periodically so that any problems can be detected, monitored, and, if necessary, treated. Urine cultures may be additionally important because they can indicate the presence of asymptomatic (no symptoms) urinary tract infections, which are common in all pregnant women.

Most women visit their obstetrician about once a month during pregnancy and possibly once a week during the last few weeks. Because you have diabetes, your physician may advise you to be examined weekly throughout your pregnancy. If you are employed, you might want to advise your employer that you will require some time off for your routine visits.

During your pregnancy your physician, nurses, and nutritionists will assist you in altering your personal care schedule to suit your daily routines. They will explain how to do your self-testing conveniently four times a day or more by the method recommended for you and how to adhere to carefully prescribed meal and snack patterns. Members of your health care team should be available every day for telephone consultations and periodically for examinations.

Second Trimester

During the second trimester the fetus undergoes its most dramatic growth. At this time the placenta (tissue connecting mother and baby) produces hormones that will cause changes in your blood sugar, and you may need to increase your insulin dosage. Some women who did not have diabetes before may become temporarily diabetic if they can't produce enough insulin. The diabetes that develops during pregnancy is called *gestational diabetes*, and it occurs because the usual hormone production is changed and sugar is not utilized as efficiently. Also, after the third month the placenta produces hormones that block the effect of insulin.

Gestational, or pregnancy, diabetes may be commonly treated with diet. When the fasting blood sugar exceeds 105 mg percent, however, insulin is necessary. If you are able to control your temporary diabetic condition with diet alone, your pregnancy will be allowed to go longer and you may not require early hospitalization as other diabetic mothers do. If the diabetes discovered during pregnancy did not exist before, it frequently will not be present after delivery. Your physician will explain to you the necessity of periodic checkups because having had diabetes during pregnancy indicates that you have an increased risk for developing diabetes later in life. Additionally, you should be sure to have a checkup for diabetes before you become pregnant again if any of the following applies to you.

- You have a family history of diabetes.
- You are over 25 years old.

- You have delivered stillborn or overweight babies.
- You have frequent yeast infections.
- You were on oral contraceptives or have ever had sugar in the urine.

If you are an insulin-dependent diabetic, as your pregnancy progresses you may find that your need for insulin doubles or even triples. This is no cause for alarm. It simply means that your pregnancy is progressing as expected. As your blood sugar rises, however, there is increased danger of ketoacidosis (diabetic coma), but if you test yourself frequently, you will be aware of any changes in your control and you can act accordingly.

When you visit your physician's office for routine examinations your medical team may recommend ultrasound techniques to be sure that your baby's growth is progressing well. Ultrasound is a technique in which sound waves are used to determine the size, position, and rate of growth of your baby and other factors concerning your pregnancy.

Third Trimester

Your physician will probably recommend additional tests during your weekly visits during the third trimester. For example, a hormone called *estriol*, produced by the fetus and the placenta, may be measured by testing either your blood or your urine. Estriol levels within normal ranges mean that mother and fetus are progressing normally. This test is frequently advised about the 30th week of the pregnancy and may be done weekly or more often until delivery.

Another test that will be explained to you by your physician at this time will be one to monitor your baby's heartbeat that is called the *non-stress* or *oxytocin challenge test*. This will be done as you lie quietly while an electrocardiogramlike machine is placed on your abdomen. The baby's heartbeat will be monitored as you lie still (nonstress) or as a substance (oxytocin) is gently inserted into your veins, causing the uterus to contract slightly. During the last weeks of pregnancy this test can alert your physician to the urgency of delivering your baby right away by its heart rate response to oxytocin.

Also in the third trimester another ultrasound test will be done, and the results will be compared with those of the first one to be sure that growth of the fetus has progressed as anticipated. If satisfactory growth has not occurred, to promote the flow of oxygen and nutrients to the baby, your physician may advise complete bed rest or other changes in your care for the remaining weeks.

Complications of Complicate Diabetes Pregnancy

If you have any complications of diabetes, you may have additional difficulties such as toxemia during your pregnancy. For example, if you have kidney disease, edema (retention of water by the tissues of your body) may be aggravated. Also, the level of protein in your urine may increase. If you had high blood pressure before, it may be even higher during pregnancy. Many diabetic women who did not have high blood pressure before may find that they have it during pregnancy.

Your physician will outline a special program of daily rest and relaxation for you if you have kidney disease or high blood pressure. If your symptoms become severe, your physician may even recommend hospitalization for a few weeks to assure that you are getting adequate rest. If you work outside your home, you may find that you have to leave your job earlier than anticipated for this reason.

Hospitalization

During your early consultations your physician will explain to your that women who have diabetes usually are hospitalized for a week or more before delivery. This is done to assure that your diabetes is under control and that any fetal difficulties can be detected before the birth process begins.

Being in the hospital will assure that your baby's activity and heart rate are being monitored carefully. You will be confident that you are only minutes away from delivery if any difficulties arise. While hospitalized before the birth you will meet other expectant mothers who also have diabetes and with whom you can share experiences and concerns.

Estriol tests may be done every day, and the nonstress test or oxytocin stress test will be done about twice a week. Your physician may recommend that you also undergo amniocentesis, a test in which a needle is inserted through the skin of your abdomen directly into the uterine cavity. A sample of amniotic fluid surrounding the fetus will be withdrawn from the uterus. When properly carried out, this test is not expected to affect the pregnancy. From the fluid, measurements of substances produced by the baby's lungs can be taken to determine whether the child's lungs are mature enough for the baby to breathe normally after delivery. Mature lungs indicate that the child will have healthy lungs at birth.

The Birth of Your Baby

Until the specialized tests were available to permit physicians to monitor your baby closely most babies of mothers with diabetes were delivered before or during the 35–37th week (normal gestational time is 40 weeks). Now it is likely that your baby can remain in your uterus longer and that the fetus will be more mature at the time of birth. While you may have heard that many women with diabetes have cesarean (surgical) deliveries, it has become more likely that you will be able to have a vaginal delivery. Your physician will discuss these possibilities with you as your pregnancy progresses. However, if this is not your first delivery, and you have had a cesarean section once or more often, you will probably deliver the same way to protect your earlier incisions. Cesarean section will also be done if the fetus is in difficulty or is mature enough for birth and labor cannot be induced.

During the first few days after the birth you will probably have a marked decrease in your insulin requirement. Within another few days, however, you will return to your prepregnancy state and will be able to return to former habits of controlling your diabetes. Women with gestational diabetes may become less insulin-dependent for an indefinite period, but insulin should not be discontinued entirely until enough time has passed to determine whether the diabetes can be controlled without it.

The Diabetic Nursing Mother

You will be advised by your physician about returning to your prepregnancy program of diet, insulin, and exercise. If you plan to nurse your baby, and physicians say that diabetic women can do so as well as nondiabetic women, you will need to raise your food intake and may need an insulin dosage adjustment. If you have gestational, or pregnancy, diabetes, you may be advised to stop taking insulin soon after delivery.

Menstruation

Young women with diabetes may notice that their patterns regarding menstruation are different from those of women who do not have diabetes. While most young women begin menstruation when they are about 12–14 years old, some women with diabetes begin as late as age 16. Women with diabetes usually begin later, especially if their diabetes is poorly controlled. Poor nutrition or an inappropriate insulin dosage can cause disturbances of hormonal balance and thus physical development.

Women with diabetes also may notice an irregularity in their monthly cycle. Improved control of the diabetes will also contribute to increased regularity of the menses.

Hormonal changes occur in all women prior to and during menstruation. For the diabetic woman these changes affect how insulin is utilized. A rise in blood sugar can occur, for example. If you have insulin-dependent diabetes, you may also have to readjust your insulin dosage or reduce food intake to counteract the possibility of higher blood sugar. During your period your estrogen and progesterone levels will vary, as will your blood sugar level. At this time you may be advised to adjust your insulin dosage. Your health care team will outline special care routines for you during your periods, which might include a slight reduction of food intake just prior to your period and possibly a slight reduction of fluid intake.

Menopause

Around age 40–50 menstruation ceases. Some women stop having periods earlier than others. Some stop suddenly while others have only a few periods a year during a several-year time span. Many think they have stopped menstruating because they have not had a period in several months or longer and then begin menstruating regularly again.

When menopause occurs, changes take place in the woman's body. Along with a decrease in the amount of estrogen and progesterone some women experience symptoms of "hot flashes," headache, and depression. A tendency toward brittle bones occurs because of the reduced amount of hormones in the body; many older women sustain fractures because of this change in their bodies. However, many women report no menopausal symptoms, and that time of life progresses as normally as other periods in their lives.

As an insulin-dependent diabetic woman, however, you may have some special concerns. For example, it may be difficult for you to distinguish menopausal hot flashes from low blood sugar reactions causing similar symptoms. If you think the hot flashes are from low blood sugar and take extra sugar or food, you may raise your blood sugar level too high. And if you think a hypoglycemic reaction is a hot flash, you may neglect to take sugar and make your low blood sugar reaction worse. To avoid this confusion, test your own blood sugar.

Other symptoms of menopause may also concern you as a diabetic if you are age 40 or over. Your blood sugar level responds to antidepressive medications as well as to mental stress. Proper relaxation and a healthy perspective on life will help you avoid undue stress and the need for antidepressant medications. Also, brittle bones are characteristic of diabetics, particularly in menopausal and postmenopausal women. Your physician may recommend that you supplement your diet with calcium-rich foods.

Sexual Activity and Contraception

Sexual activity can be energy-expending. If you are sexually active and have insulin-dependent diabetes, you will want to remember to have additional glucose in the form of nutritional snacks available for use around the time of such activity, especially if it takes place at a time of diminished food intake and continued insulin availability, such as late at night, early in the morning, or before meals.

Most physicians advise women who have diabetes to have any children they want while they are young; they suggest that up to age 30 is the optimal period. Women who have diabetes usually are advised not to use oral contraceptives because they may adversely affect metabolism or accelerate vascular disease. Most doctors advise diabetic women to use other methods, such as an intrauterine device or diaphragm.

As a woman with diabetes, you can plan to enjoy a normal life cycle. With supervision from your physician and health care team and appropriate control of your disease, your life can be filled with joys and enrichment.

7

Diabetic Children

If your child has diabetes, he or she can continue to lead a normal childhood, attend regular schools, go to summer camp, travel, and participate in athletic activities. You can let your child continue to be a child. When the disease is under control and the child is knowledgeable about diabetes strenuous activities are not harmful. Many professional athletes have diabetes.

Diabetes is not contagious. There is no way one child can "catch it" from another. And, unlike most of the illnesses the child has had before, diabetes is a disorder that rarely goes away by itself. Early recognition and treatment of the disease are important. The goal of treatment will be adequate growth for the child, both physical and mental. You, your child, and other family members will want to learn as much as possible about living with diabetes so that family life can continue as smoothly as possible.

Causes of Juvenile Diabetes

Your child will probably ask many questions about diabetes, just as you will. Why your child? The causes of diabetes in young children and adolescents are not known. Heredity plays a role, but heredity alone is not enough to cause diabetes. According to the American Diabetes Association, recent research indicates that certain viruses may combine with an inherited susceptibility and play a role in the development of diabetes. Of the 15 million Indians who have diabetes, many cases began in childhood or adolescence. A child's diabetes is not the result of anything the parents do or do not do.

If your child is old enough, he or she will be able to understand that diabetes is a condition in which the body doesn't utilize food appropriately because of the lack of insulin, the hormone produced in the pancreas. The lack of insulin causes sugar (in the form of glucose) to build up in the blood and urine. It isn't distributed throughout the body to produce energy as it should.

You may have noticed that your child was weak, was constantly thirsty and hungry, and urinated frequently. Many cases of diabetes in children under age 15 appear suddenly. Unlike non-insulin-dependent diabetes, which is often related to obesity in adults, diabetes in children has little to do with weight. While losing weight may contribute to your diabetic child's comfort and self-esteem, the weight loss alone probably will not be enough to stabilize the blood sugar level. If your child's case is like many of the juvenile-onset type, it is very likely to be insulin-dependent and will require daily insulin injections.

Your child may be admitted to a hospital after the diagnosis is made so that additional tests can be performed and the optimal level of insulin can be prescribed and monitored for a few days. Your learning process and the child's learning process will begin at that time. You will both learn how to function at home within the family structure and, if the child is old enough, how to feel secure with self-care.

The health care team's educational approach and care plan for your young child with diabetes will be geared to encourage independence. Your physician will strive to preserve your child's previous lifestyle as much as possible and center the diet and insulin needs around it. For example, if your child is sports-minded, athletic activities will not have to be curtailed if the child has fairly good control of the disease. With an older child the health care team's goal will be to enable the child to assume responsibility for injections and insulin measurement, diet, and self-monitoring without being totally dependent on you or the doctor.

The health care team will work with you to help you combat any tendencies toward overprotectiveness and possible guilt concerning your child's disease. You will learn to cope with your child's adaptation to regulation and new sense of discipline necessary to control the disease properly. Health care professionals will be available to provide advice, instructional materials, and emotional support for you.

Coping with Your Diabetic Child

As you learn to help your child regulate his or her body chemistry for a healthier life, remember to do what your physician and health care team advise. Friends and relatives will offer well-meaning advice and suggestions that may be based on something they read or heard and may or may not be applicable to your child's condition. Control of your child's diabetes will depend on proper diet, emotional stability, well-regulated insulin injections, exercise, and regular glucose testing. (See Chapter 8 for more information on self-testing.)

Families that have adjusted well to caring for a diabetic child do not make the child's diabetes a central concern to the family and do not need to change the entire family's lifestyle. If you set reasonable goals for diet, testing, exercise, and self-care, your child will adapt to the situation with flexibility and good humor, and so will others in the family.

The best assistance you can give your child or adolescent with diabetes is to keep calm and not express constant concern over every detail of the management of the diabetes. Your matter-of-fact attitude will rub off on your child. If you accept the additional activities of daily living related to diabetic care as part of the family routine, so will your child. Your child should come to view diabetic care as an uncomplicating and uncomplicated aspect of life.

If your child takes injections, he will learn to view the minor discomfort as part of his regular day, just as he accepts daily hygiene routines, occasional skinned knees, falls from his bicycle, and other cuts and bruises. If you express too much sympathy for occasional discomfort, your child may begin to feel sorry for himself and thus have a harder time taking the injections and caring for himself.

Children with diabetes should not be permitted to use their disease as a frequent excuse for avoiding special lessons, taking the school bus, or other situations. Of course, occasional headaches or sick spells may occur just as they do in nondiabetic children. However, you should encourage the diabetic child to learn to view illness as something to overcome, not something to hide behind. If you, as the parent, are not overprotective and encourage carrying on routine activities despite some occasional under-par feelings, your child will develop a mature outlook toward living with diabetes.

Encourage your child to follow his or her physician's recommendations to take the daily injections of insulin at the same time each day, using the correct dosage. A common cause of poor diabetic control is changing the time of day for the injection and taking an incorrect dose of the injection. Frequent and unnecessary changes may cause blood sugar to become too low and then go too high.

Additionally your doctor may recommend that you do not adjust the amount of insulin on days when your child expects more activity than usual. Instead, you can give the child additional food before he or she engages in heavy sports activities. Also, the child may keep some extra food handy in case of an insulin reaction (low blood sugar) during a game or strenuous activity.

Overall, your role in coping with your diabetic child will be supportive but should not be overindulgent. Encourage self-care and participation in routine activities. However, two medical emergencies may require quick action on your part: hypoglycemia (low blood sugar) and ketoacidosis (diabetic coma). There may be times when you suspect that either of these reactions is taking place. If you suspect low blood sugar, use a self-monitoring blood glucose test, if you can. Or use a urine test for acetone, a sign of possible ketoacidosis. Ketones do not always indicate ketoacidosis, as it may result from emotional stress, diet, exercise, and especially low blood sugar. Your health care team will give you specific instructions to follow if these condtions occur.

How Much Should a Diabetic Child Eat?

Each child is different. Each child's needs differ from day to day. Children who seem to eat too much may be taking more insulin than they need, and the extra insulin causes increased hunger. However, hunger can also be a signal that the blood sugar is low. You can do a blood test at the time the child is hungry. If the blood sugar level is often low, discuss changing the dosage of insulin with the doctor and nutritionist.

Diabetic children are like all children. They will want to snack between meals. For a diabetic child being treated with insulin, calculated snacking is important because the injected insulin continues to work even if no food is eaten. If a child's meal is delayed for any reason, a snack should be given and then the meal should be reduced in size. Appropriate snacks for a diabetic child are ones with nutritional value, such as cheese, crackers, peanut butter, and skim milk. Raisins and other dried fruits are also good snacks for the child to carry with him or her.

Playtime and Exercise

Children get exercise during playtime. They run and jump and often engage in vigorous activities such as bicycling, tennis, and football. Exercise is a natural part of childhood and is essential to control diabetes. During exercise the child burns up sugar, thus decreasing his need for insulin. His circulation will improve, and with sufficient exercise the likelihood of becoming overweight will decrease.

Your physician will question you and your child about diet and exercise habits and may change the recommended food intake according to the amount of exercise the child gets. For a child who exercises strenuously, as in playing tennis or football, the physician may recommend extra food for needed energy or special snacks before a game to prevent low blood sugar. Also, your physician may change the dose of insulin to allow for the extra exercise.

Self-Care by Your Child

How much responsibility for diabetes self-care that children will accept varies from individual to individual and, of course, depends on age. A two- or three-year-old is not ready to assume responsibility for self-care but can participate in activities initiated by parents, such as planning a snack based on choices presented by parents. At age four to six the child will need reinforcement of his strengths, as he realizes that he is a little different from his nondiabetic friends. At this age the child will begin to understand that an insulin reaction may occur unless he eats prior to exercising. At age seven to eight, though not likely to fully comprehend the reasons for treatment, the child can learn to handle simple self-care, such as measuring or even administering insulin. Around age 9 to 11 many diabetic children can manage their own insulin injections and urine testing. Some children are ready to do their own insulin injections earlier than others. Some are more adept with their fingers than others. When the child expresses interest in administering his own injections you should plan to supervise the procedure. Your health care team will advise you of "practice" procedures for your child to learn injection techniques, such as injecting water into an orange or apple.

By the time the child is about 12 he can probably make some decisions for himself. For example, he will understand the possible consequences of skipping his insulin. When the child is a little older he should be able to manage self-care entirely. At this age children should also receive information on the effects of alcohol and drug substances (such as marijuana) as well as on contraception and pregnancy. Children may prefer to monitor their blood sugar levels instead of using the urine test. Also, blood tests give a clearer picture of control because they give exact measures of blood sugar (see Chapter 8).

What Parents and School Personnel Need to Know

Coping with Reactions

Diabetic children attend regular schools. However, you should inform the teaching staff of your child's condition and determine whether they know the essentials of diabetic management.

The school personnel should be able to recognize any behavioral changes that may signal an insulin reaction or low blood sugar. They should be aware of the sudden onset of pallor, sweating, sudden hunger, poor coordination, and disorientation. This can happen as a result of missed meals or failure to eat before strenuous exercise. The treatment is to provide sugar in the form of any food or drink, such as fruit juice or candy. If the child doesn't feel better in 10-15 minutes, he should be taken to a hospital, or a paramedical team should be called if one is available in the community. Some physicians train the family and school personnel in use of glucagon for insulin shock.

High blood sugar is a less common reaction, but it may require prompt medical attention. This type of reaction comes on gradually. Signs are drowsiness, extreme thirst, frequent urination, flushed skin, vomiting, fruity breath odor and heavy breathing, and possibly loss of consciousness. This can happen as a result of not taking insulin or of stress, illness, injury, or too much food or drink. A child with high blood sugar should contact his or her health care team or be taken to a hospital.

How can you or school personnel tell whether the reaction is low blood sugar or high blood sugar? Possibly the child can state what he or she has or has not done to cause the attack. Also, you may try to give the child some food or drink containing sugar. If that doesn't help within a few minutes, or if the child cannot take anything by mouth, he probably needs medical attention and paramedics should be called, or the child should be taken to a hospital for treatment.

School Schedules

School personnel should know about the child's daily plan for balancing diet, exercise, and insulin. You can provide school personnel with information about the child's daily dietary requirements. You should advise the teacher, for example, if between-meal snacks are or are not part of the daily plan. Children who have to test urine or blood for sugar level before lunch should be permitted to leave the classroom for this purpose. Finally, school personnel should know how to reach you and the physician at all times. Scheduling of meals and physical education classes should be discussed with school personnel and the physician.

Eating Away From Home

All children love to go to parties, visit friends overnight, and travel. If your child is going to a friend's house, you can help him maintain his diabetic control by encouraging him to plan ahead. For instance, he may want to discuss special-occasion eating with his doctor. Also, he may want to ask the friend's parent to provide artificially sweetened beverages or ice cream for him. He may want to bring some of his own refreshments. He will want to explain the need for timing of meals to an adult at the friend's house and plan the menu to avoid embarrassment.

A teenager will be able to adjust his or her own diet so that occasional eating out with friends can be enjoyed.

Travelling

You can obtain a special insulated travel kit for storing your child's supplies of insulin. It should be kept in a cool place but not necessarily in the refrigerator. Your child should also carry a letter or prescription from his or her doctor for an insulin syringe and needle in case the kit is lost. Most states require prescriptions for hypodermic equipment. You child should carry snacks with available glucose and continue to test routinely, just as he would do at home. If an emergency need for equipment or a physician arises while away from home, you can contact the local affiliated chapter of the American Diabetes Association or the nearest hospital or medical society.

Diabetic children can go to summer camp. In fact, many health care teams encourage young patients to attend special camps geared toward teaching diabetic children to care for themselves. Many recommend that the first visit be arranged soon after diagnosis. They say that meeting other children with the same problem can assist the child to accept his condition and encourage him to make new friends. These camps also provide healthful recreation and a wide variety of sports activities and are often sponsored by the American Diabetes Association.

Once the child has the diabetes under control, he or she may attend some regular summer camps. However, the camp directors and counselors, just as teachers in school, should be aware of the child's diabetic condition and demonstrate the capability to handle the diabetic child. Adequate supplies of diabetic equipment should be provided for the child's use at camp, whether it is a special camp or a camp for nondiabetic children.

The Joys of Parenting

Being a parent of a diabetic child gives you a special responsibility. While you may be aware of the complications that can occur as a result of diabetes, parents of diabetic youngsters say it is best if you do not express your fears to your child but educate him or her about the advantages of diabetic control. Not all diabetics have complications of their disease. Only a relatively small percentage of diabetics have kidney disease or visual difficulties. Treatments for these complications continue to improve, and if your child should develop any of these as a result of diabetes, the outlook for management is good. The important thing to remember is that a consistently positive attitude on your part will assist your child in accepting the fact that his personal care includes some aspects that are a little different from his nondiabetic friends' routines.

Your overall relationship with your child and how you speak about his handling of his disease may also have an effect on his self-care performance. For example, if you show interest in all his activities and schoolwork as well as his general well-being, rather than just his diabetes, you will encourage him to think of his special routines as part of everyday life rather than as a problem. Make the child aware of diabetics who have handled the disease well and functioned in a normal manner. Seek help from competent health care professionals in diabetes and the support of your local diabetes association as well as community and hospital support groups.

Parenting a diabetic child has its joys, too. You will take pride in seeing your child adapt to the special routines of care. You will feel good when your child feels good. A few extra hugs and words of praise will be in order on many occasions. To the treatment plan of diet, insulin, and exercise, add a little love.

8

Self-Monitoring Diabetes

Because control of your diabetes depends mostly on a balance of diet, exercise, insulin, and emotions, daily self-monitoring of your control of your disease may be recommended by your physician. Through careful monitoring you and your physician can determine any need for adjustments in these keys to your good health. The benefits of self-monitoring vary among individuals, and your physician will explain how the merits of various tests relate to you and your condition.

If you have insulin-dependent diabetes, your doctor will probably ask you to test your glucose level several times throughout each day. The goal will be to obtain consistently normal results. If you detect a change, you will be asked to watch to see if any pattern is developing. Depending on the situation, your doctor may recommend that you vary your insulin dosage, alter your diet or exercise program, or make an office visit.

Self-testing is particularly valuable for patients with "brittle" or unstable diabetes who have wide swings in blood sugar levels. It is also helpful for those who have complications of diabetes, such as kidney or eye problems.

If your before-meal readings are consistently normal, your doctor may have you begin with readings after meals, a time when glucose levels are more likely to be high. If these readings are consistently normal, you may then be advised to test less frequently.

Home glucose monitoring can be very useful for patients who cannot always tell whether or not they are experiencing hypoglycemia (low blood sugar). Such patients may often misjudge their situation and take simple carbohydrates in an attempt to raise a blood sugar level that is actually already normal. As a response to this, their blood sugar continues to rise. In such cases, if the patients tested their blood sugar first, they would discover that they were not hypoglycemic and could avoid causing unnecessarily high blood sugar and poor control.

During pregnancy self-testing is particularly important because diabetic control can greatly reduce the number of fetal abnormalities and stillbirths among infants of diabetic mothers.

In patients treated only by diet or by diet and oral medication, home monitoring may be less necessary because blood glucose levels fluctuate less.

Self-Testing with a Blood Sample

Your physician and health care team will acquaint you with the various products available with which you can test your blood for glucose level. They will explain techniques that will be easy to follow. And they will make specific recommendations so that your testing routine will fit into your daily routine.

Your self-testing procedure will involve pricking your finger to draw a drop of blood. Convenient pricking devices are available nis purpose. You will then transfer the drop of blood to a tiny strip with a chemically coated pad at one end, wait one minute, and watch the pad change color according to the amount of glucose present in your blood. With some strips you can compare the color with colors on a chart and estimate your blood sugar by matching colors visually. With other strips the end of the strip is inserted into a metering device, which displays a digital readout of your blood sugar level. Metering devices are small enough to tuck into a purse or briefcase.

Physicians say there is little difference in accuracy between the two methods. However, people who have visual impairments often have more success using the digital readout device than with the visual comparison method. Metering devices are more expensive, however, ranging in price to several hundred dollars. Still, the largest part of the expense in the long range is in the cost of the test strips. They range in cost markedly by type and by area in which they are purchased. Comparative price shopping is recommended. Your physician and health care team will advise you on ways to purchase your testing strips in quantity and may advise slicing strips lengthwise and thus obtaining two for the price of one, if accuracy can be maintained that way. Some of the strips retain their color in their container and can be labeled and checked for accurate readings with your health care team.

Self-Testing with a Urine Sample

Several urine tests are available for monitoring glucose level with a urine specimen. Your health care team will select the one most appropriate for you and will advise you on how many times a day to test your urine. For example, if you are insulin-dependent, you will probably be asked to test before each meal and at bedtime. If acceptable blood tests are done, urine tests may not be necessary.

Your health care team will explain several factors that you should understand concerning the validity of self-monitored urine tests. One is your *renal threshold*, the blood sugar level at which your kidneys spill excess glucose from your bloodstream into your urine. Renal thresholds vary among individuals. They usually are higher in older adults. The normal renal threshold for most middle-aged people is 160–180 mg of sugar per deciliter of blood. Thus a person whose renal threshold is higher than 200 mg/dl may not find urine testing helpful because it does not dependably reflect the blood sugar, and the person may not be aware of poor control. Some patients may have low thresholds, as during pregnancy. Then the blood sugar test is recommended.

Some people test "first-voided" specimens. Others test "second-voided" specimens. Your health care team will explain that the first-voided sample indicates diabetic control over a period of several hours with urine collected in the bladder; the second-voided sample indicates level of control at the moment. The kind of sample you test can make a difference in what you do about the results.

Some urine tests for use at home or while traveling involve placing a few drops of urine in a test tube and adding water and a tablet containing a special preparation designed to react to the glucose component of the urine. After 15 seconds you compare the color of the test tube liquid with those on a color chart.

Other urine tests involve dipping a small strip or stick into the urine, waiting 15 seconds for a reaction to take place, and comparing color changes.

Blood Testing Versus Urine Testing

How can you determine whether to use blood or urine tests for your self-monitoring at home? Your physician will advise you of the merits of both methods and techniques. Generally, however, most physicians believe that blood tests provide a more accurate picture of blood glucose levels than urine tests. This is because urine is retained in the bladder for hours before it is tested, while your blood is constantly circulating and reacting to your body chemistry. A blood test will give you a more immediate reading of your glucose level.

Blood sugar tests can enable you to make careful adjustments to maintain blood sugar at a level as close as possible to normal. This is particularly important if you are pregnant; if you have frequently occurring insulin reactions, kidney disease, or a high renal threshold; and during illness. Also, blood testing is recommended for infants who are not toilet-trained.

Tips on Testing Materials

When your health care team provides you with instructions regarding self-monitoring, they will also give you some helpful hints for becoming more efficient about the testing procedures as well as saving money. For example, they will advise you on where to purchase your equipment and what quantity to buy. Health professionals learn this kind of consumer information from other diabetics and will be happy to share it with you. Diabetics have found it helpful, for instance, always to check the expiration dates on equipment. Also, directions for timing various tests differ. You should remember to check and follow timing directions carefully because timing is essential to getting accurate results. And, when recording your test results, remember that percentages, pluses, and minuses may not read the same with all tests.

As you begin your self-monitoring procedures your health care team will be available to answer questions. Your questions are probably like those of most other diabetics, and a few helpful answers at the right time will be essential to put you on the right track.

Why Self-Monitor?

Should you monitor your glucose level yourself? Physicians caring for diabetics say "yes." They say the advantages outweigh the small degree of inconvenience. Maintaining normal blood glucose helps build resistance to infection and helps prevent the possible complications associated with diabetes, including kidney, eye, and nerve disease. Evidence supports this attitude. Home glucose monitoring is a fairly recent development. The first tests were available for consumer use in the early 1970s. Since that time there have been fewer diabetic complications, and more diabetics have control of their disease because they have daily (or more frequent) readings of their glucose level and do not have to depend solely on visits to their physicians' offices for this information.

You can also self-monitor for ketones in your urine. This is especially important for juvenile diabetics, during pregnancy, and during severe stress or illness. A variety of materials is available for this purpose, including powders, tablets, and sticks. Your health care team will recommend the type of test that will be best for you to use as well as when and how to use it.

9
Living with Diabetes

Diabetes is a disease in which your personal role in your treatment has an important effect on the quality of your life. Your health care team will give you guidelines to follow for personal routines that can help you enjoy a more normal life.

As a diabetic you will want to devote a little more attention to some of your personal care than you may have done before. Your health care team will provide you with specific hints concerning care of your skin, feet, and teeth. Maintaining good skin-cleaning habits can help your skin remain healthy and protect your body effectively. Promptly treating minor injuries such as burns, cuts, and bruises helps your skin heal properly and avoids problems. Your health care team will explain that, because decreased circulation in many diabetics is often noticed first in the legs and feet, attention to foot care can help you maintain good function. Avoiding poor diabetic control can help you avoid other problems such as vascular system difficulties, kidney disease, and eye difficulties.

Your health care team will also instruct you about general hygiene, what to do when you are ill, what to do when traveling and eating out, what to do about social drinking (if you are permitted to do so at all by your physician), as well as addressing sexual concerns. If you are elderly, your health care team will tell you about special arrangements for your home health care.

Your family's emotional adjustment to your diabetes will also be an important concern which your health care team will discuss with you and members of your family. Your family's health education should begin right away. Family members will quickly learn that diabetes isn't contagious and isn't transmitted by any kind of physical contact. As you and your family learn to live with diabetes, you will all become familiar with common acute and chronic complications and their possible prevention, how to recognize circumstances warranting a call to your health care team, skills such as blood and/or urine testing, and, if necessary, injection techniques. Your health care team will assist you in living comfortably with your disease by providing continuing education during each visit.

Skin Care

Because diabetes can cause changes in the tiny blood vessels that supply your skin with nutrients, proper skin care is especially important in preventing bacterial and fungal infections, impaired nerve sensations, dry, itchy skin, and other skin disorders. Your health care team will suggest daily guidelines for your personal hygiene. These may include the following.

- After bathing, keep your skin dry, particularly in the skin folds in the armpits, the groin, and under the breasts. Use talcum powder to help yourself stay dry.
- When bathing, avoid excessively hot water and use a superfatted soap to lubricate your skin. Try to avoid harsh and highly perfumed soaps.
- Use a humidifier at home to moisten the air during the cold winter months. Use a lubricating skin oil to moisturize your skin when the humidity is low.
- Take care of any injuries to hands or feet right away. People with impaired nerve sensations tend to be more susceptible to infections, particularly in the legs and feet. Seek professional assistance for changes such as pressure injuries from shoes or changes in color of your skin and proper management of open

wounds, should they occur. Check your feet frequently, since you may not feel an injury to your feet as readily with diabetic nerve changes that create decreased sensation.

5. Avoid excessive exposure to the sun, as these burns can be serious to a diabetic because of infection, dehydration, and altered diabetic control.

Foot Care

You feel as good as your feet feel. To keep your feet feeling good, your health care team will recommend many of the following routines for you.

- After daily bathing, dry your feet well. Excessive moisture can set the scene for fungus infections, blisters, and other irritations.

- When choosing shoes and socks, be sure they fit well and do not cause pressure effects such as corns and calluses or constriction by elastic.

- Keep your toenails trimmed straight across and not too short. Avoid cutting into the corners, which could injure the soft tissue and permit infection to develop. To prevent ingrown toenails you might want to round the corners gently.

- If you do develop corns and calluses, careful use of pressure-relieving pads may help. If you want to reduce corns and calluses, discuss this with your health care team. They may recommend use of a pumice stone. If corns and calluses cause persistent pain, redness, or swelling, you will want to seek professional advice from competent specialists recommended by your medical advisors.

- If excessive dryness or cracking of the skin on your feet is a problem for you, moisturizing bath oil or skin lubricants may be helpful.

- In cold climates, wear adequate protective outer footwear. Boots should be warm, waterproof, and fitted carefully to prevent constriction, excessive rubbing, and frostbite.

- Use caution when going barefoot at swimming pools, on the

beach, and in locker rooms. Wear clogs or waterproof sandals whenever possible in public places. Wearing slippers or shoes at all times can help prevent foot injuries at home. Wear socks or stockings to absorb moisture as bare feet in moist shoes may result in blisters.

- Apply cleansing or antiseptic solutions to any openings in the skin. Call your health care team for advice if you have an injury.

Eye Care

Blood vessels in the eyes may show effects of diabetes. Your physician will probably examine your eyes during most routine visits to check for subtle changes. Additionally, to preserve your vision there are several things you can remember to do:

- Have your eyes and vision checked periodically by an ophthalmologist. If you wear glasses, be sure your prescription is up to date.
- If you notice that your vision is blurred or changed markedly, consult your physician, as diabetes control changes as well as other conditions can be treated early.
- When you have your eyes checked regularly by an ophthalmologist, be sure to make known the fact that you have diabetes. If there are signs of diabetic changes, your ophthalmologist or retinal specialist may advise a test known as an *angiogram*. With this test a dye is injected into your arm, and pictures are taken of your eyes to indicate blood vessel changes. Early treatment of these vascular changes with laser or other techniques has been extremely important in preventing progressive eye changes that occur in longtime diabetics.
- Wear protective eyewear while manipulating machinery that may cause flying particles. Wear sunglasses while outdoors in bright sunlight.
- Don't rub your eyes unnecessarily. If you have to touch your face to shave, apply makeup, or remove foreign objects from your eye, be sure your hands are clean.

- Avoid straining your eyes. Try to maintain adequate lighting when reading, writing, or working. Get enough sleep.

Dental Care

Oral hygiene is an important aspect of overall diabetic care. Your teeth and mouth tissues must be in good health to prevent dental problems that could have serious complications, such as gingivitis. To keep your mouth in top condition your health care team will recommend that you follow a few suggestions:

- See your dentist at least twice a year. Have a checkup and have your teeth cleaned (prophylaxis) at least twice a year. Follow your dentist's recommendations for mouth x-rays, which will permit changes in bony structures to be seen.
- Brush your teeth regularly, at least twice a day, following instructions from your dentist or oral hygienist. If possible, keep a toothbrush in your purse or pocket so that you can brush during your workday or while away from home after meals. Floss your teeth daily according to your dentist's recommendations.
- If any scratches, sores, or other injuries appear in your mouth, seek professional advice. Avoid using too-hard toothbrushes that might irritate delicate oral tissue.
- Be sure to tell your dentist that you have diabetes. Your dental office may wish to contact your health care team before any dental procedures are done.

Travel

Travel is part of the spice of life. A little change of scene is as good for diabetics as for nondiabetics. Along with a change of scene, however, comes a change in personal care routines. As a diabetic you should plan for changes in your routine ahead of time by consulting your health care team. Plan as far ahead as possible. Learn the locations of local American Diabetes Association affiliates in the areas in which you will travel. Other suggestions your health care team may make include the following.

- Carry enough supplies with you so that, if you stay away longer than you originally plan, you won't have to look for supplies (especially important in foreign countries).
- In a separate case, carry your urine and/or blood testing equipment as well as insulin, syringes, and swabs. Don't pack these items in luggage that you check on a plane, train, or bus.
- Carry identification indicating that you have diabetes and information about your medication and dosages. Carry a prescription from your doctor for your insulin and syringes. Carry antinausea medication as well as medication to relieve possible vomiting and diarrhea.
- Plan to alter your meal plan according to your travel plans. For example, when traveling by car, plan on having extra food supplies with you to avoid an insulin reaction. You can keep hard candy, raisins, graham crackers, or fruit handy.
- Store your insulin in a cool place such as inside the car with you rather than in a trunk or glove compartment, where it might be extremely warm or exposed to heat or sun.
- If you are flying, be prepared to change your insulin injection procedure if you need to have an insulin injection while in the air. Plan on putting about half the usual amount of air into your insulin bottle to balance for pressure in the cabin in a high-altitude flight.
- Be aware of changing time zones and administer your insulin injections and have your meals on your home time rather than according to the time zone you are in. Your health care team will assist you in planning ahead for time zone changes of two hours or more.
- Because traveling causes special stresses, it will be important to continue testing your glucose levels frequently to be sure that your diabetes is under control. If you notice high sugar readings, try to exercise more and reduce your intake of carbohydrates. Your health care team will give you instructions to follow regarding changes in insulin doses if your glucose level can't be controlled with exercise and carbohydrates.
- Be careful about getting blisters from more walking than usual. Try to break in new shoes before going on a trip. If you do get

a blister on your foot, try to keep the blister from breaking by covering it with a simple dressing. Don't use tapes that injure the skin further. Use paper or special tape. Your health care team will advise you about various first aid procedures for such injuries.

- Learn to say (or carry a card with you reading) "I have diabetes" in the languages spoken in the area in which you might travel.

- Tell your traveling companion(s) that you are diabetic and how they can assist you in case you need help. If you are on a tour, be sure that the tour guide or operator knows about your special needs, particularly about having meals at proper intervals and about what to do if a medical emergency occurs.

Eating Out

Eating out can be fun for you as well as your companions. The difference is that you, as a diabetic, will want to remember to fit your eating out into your overall meal plan and allotted exchanges for each day. You will want to be careful to keep high-sugar foods to a minimum and avoid highly salted foods. Watch portion sizes so that you do not unknowingly consume too many calories during one meal.

When preparing your meal plan your health care team will ask questions about your eating out habits and make some general recommendations for you to use as guidelines when you eat out. Following are some tips.

- Become familiar with your meal plan. Know it well. If you can't remember it all, carry a copy with you. Become familiar with foods and portion sizes on your exchange lists.

- Ask questions about how food is prepared before you order it. Try to advise your hosts or the restaurants you patronize that you have diabetes to avoid meal delays and inappropriate meals.

- When you know that there will be a wait for a table in a restaurant or at a group meal, such as a banquet, carry a snack to eat while waiting but then plan to eliminate part of the meal to account for the snack in your total daily caloric intake.

- Ask local restaurant owners to provide more menu variety, more salad bars, and better beverage choices. Be a strong consumer and make your desires and needs known.
- Ask for substitutions in restaurants. If inappropriate foods are part of the meal, ask for another food in their place or simply skip some foods but maintain the calories and balance of your meal.
- Choose foods that are not prepared with sauces or gravies. Try to avoid breaded or creamed dishes; they are likely to be higher in calories than plainer foods.

How About a Drink?

Guidelines

1. Discuss the use of alcohol with your physician.
2. Do not drink on an empty stomach.
3. Drink slowly.
4. Avoid sugary, sweet drinks.
5. Make the necessary caloric adjustments to compensate for the alcoholic beverage.
6. If you drink, do it in moderation (never to the point that judgment is impaired).

If you are accustomed to having an occasional alcoholic drink, you may want to ask your physician about the timing of such beverages and the types you can drink safely. Many physicians say it is not harmful for most people with diabetes whose disease is under control to have a drink once in a while. However, remember that alcohol consumed before or during a meal may produce changes in your blood sugar. Alcohol drunk before a meal may cause a drop in your blood sugar. Since alcohol consumed must be calculated into your daily caloric intake, be aware of the caloric content of your favorite drinks (see Table 9-1). In younger persons with diabetes parental supervision will

Table 7
Whiskey, Wine and Beer Caloric and Exchange Details*

	Serving Size	Approximate Calories	Number of Exchanges
Distilled Whiskey (86 Proof)	45 gms	107	2½ fat
Dry Table Wine (12% alcohol)	90 gms	68	1½ fat
Regular Beer (4.5% alcohol)	360 gms	151	3½ fat or 2 fat & 1 Bread
"Light" Beer (3.5% alcohol)	360 gms	97	2 fat

*Source : American Diabetes Association.

Table 8
Alcoholic Beverages Containing No Carbohydrate*

Beverage	Amount	Exchange
Beer (Light)	360 gms	2 fat
Cocktails (Freshly made)		
Highball 1½ oz. distilled spirit and water, club soda, or diet soft drink	340 gms	2 fat
Martini 1½ oz. dry gin, ½ oz. dry vermouth	105 gms	3 fat
Cocktails (Premixed)		
Martini	105 gms	4 fat
Vodka Martini	105 gms	4 fat
Distilled Spirits (86 proof)		
Brandy	30 gms	2 fat
Bourbon	30 gms	2 fat
Cognac	30 gms	2 fat

* The exchanges are based on the use of 86 proof distilled spirits when used in any of the previous recipes.

Alcoholic Beverages Containing No Carbohydrate (cont.)

Beverage	Amount	Exchange
Distilled Spirits (86 proof)		
Canadian whiskey	30 gms	2 fat
Gin	30 gms	2 fat
Rye	30 gms	2 fat
Rum	30 gms	2 fat
Scotch	30 gms	2 fat
Tequila	30 gms	2 fat
Vodka	30 gms	2 fat
Liqueurs, Cordials		
Akvavit	30 gms	1 fat
Ginger-flavored brandy	30 gms	2 fat
Kümmel	30 gms	2 fat
Southern Comfort	30 gms	3 fat
Wines		
Champagne	30 gms	2 fat
Red table wine, dry	30 gms	2 fat
Sauterne	105 gms	2 fat
Sherry, dry	90 gms	3 fat
White table wine, dry	90 gms	2 fat
Mixes		
Club soda	300 gms	Free

play a role in consumption of alcoholic beverages. Parents may wish to make their own family habits regarding this matter known to the child's physician. In some cases alcohol use by persons with diabetes or abuse of alcohol can have serious consequences. If you have been a heavy drinker, you might want to discuss your habits with your health care team, which will assist you in trying to alter your habit to fit the requirements of your dietary therapy for your diabetes.

Also, if you have non-insulin-dependent diabetes and take one of the oral hypoglycemics, alcohol may cause extreme flushing, and you may notice a very warm sensation and some redness of the skin.

If your diabetes is out of control, consumption of alcoholic beverages should be avoided.

Your health care team will give you some general guidelines, from which you can draw the aspects that are most applicable to you. These may include the following.

- If you have certain forms of heart or kidney disease, gastritis (inflammation of the stomach) or pancreatitis (inflammation of the pancreas), you will probably be advised to avoid drinking. Also, if you have high triglyceride levels (certain fats in the blood), you will probably be advised to avoid drinking. Chronic consumption of alcohol can aggravate the condition, which in turn may be a major cause of atherosclerosis.

- If you are not eating regularly, drinking can produce hypoglycemia because alcohol taken while fasting enhances the blood sugar action of insulin and interferes with your body's ability to produce glucose.

- If you are taking oral glucose-lowering medications, alcohol can cause a lowering of your blood sugar.

- If you are dieting to lose weight, remember that alcohol provides calories but has little nutritional value. Alcohol should contribute no more than 6 percent of your total calories each day.

- Alcoholic drinks are usually calculated as fat exchanges. Check your meal plan and omit appropriate fat exchanges for the day if you have had a drink. If you cook with alcohol, you do not have to calculate the amounts you use in your meal plan because the alcohol evaporates as it cooks. Few calories remain, making alcohol a good low-calorie flavoring.

- It may be helpful to know that dry wines usually contain moderate amounts of alcohol (12 percent) and have little or no sugar. Very sweet dessert wines and liqueurs have up to 50 percent sugar and should be avoided.

- Keep in mind the dangers of mixing alcohol and medications. You may want to talk to your physician or pharmacist about

the advisability of drinking while taking certain prescriptions or over-the-counter medications.
• Remember that alcohol dependency is generally unhealthy for diabetics and nondiabetics. Alcohol can damage all the vital organs in the body.

Make the Best of Sick Days

Most people have days when they feel a little under par. Diabetics and nondiabetics alike get colds, flu, upset stomachs, and other common ailments. When this happens, rest, relax, and make the best of the day. However, keep in mind that, as a diabetic, these minor ailments can be more serious for you than for others because illnesses of any kind can temporarily interrupt your control of your disease.

Illness of any type promotes stress, and stress in turn can raise your blood sugar level and cause a loss of control. If you are unable to eat or drink because of illness, you will learn to make certain adjustments in your insulin therapy. At some times you will be able to make these adjustments yourself without calling your physician. At other times you will want to seek professional advice. Self-monitoring of your glucose level will be important at such times, and when you call your physician you may be asked about the results of your at-home tests. Some specifics to remember regarding sick days are:

• Keep your physician's phone number handy. Know how to reach other members of the health care team. Be sure others in your family also have these phone numbers.
• Ask your physician and health care team to prepare a sick-day menu plan for you during one of your routine visits. They will give you several variations of your regular menu plan to follow when you do not feel well.
• Carefully record results of your home urine and/or blood tests. Do not omit your home tests, especially if you do not feel well. Also record your fluid and food intake so that you can report these to your doctor when you call on a sick day.

- Take your usual dose of insulin. If your self-tests are high for sugar, test for ketones; if ketones are present, call your doctor right away. You may need extra insulin.
- Report vomiting episodes to your doctor right away. Keep available an antiemetic prescribed for you to control nausea and vomiting and use it according to your physician's directions.
- If you are ill, your doctor's advice may be to stay in bed for a few days, drink plenty of liquids, and take medication as advised. Your health care team will make individual recommendations to help you keep your diabetes under control. You should notify them when you are ill so that adjustments in your routine can be made.
- If you have a bacterial infection and your physician prescribes an antibiotic medication for you, be sure to take it according to directions. Antibiotics will not interfere with your diabetic control.

If you have to be hospitalized, you will have some special nutritional needs. For example, if you require surgery, you might be advised to consume more calories than usual for a while to build up your strength. At this time your physician may adjust your insulin dosage to accommodate for the extra food. Your diabetes health care team will work closely with your general or specialized surgeon to adjust techniques such as anesthesia and medications to meet your specific needs at this time.

Care of Elderly Diabetics

Some older persons with diabetes find the routines of their diabetic care stressful and sometimes fail to comply with recommendations for control of their disease. If you have an older relative in your household who requires special attention to diabetic control, you can be supportive by reinforcing the physician's instructions, emphasizing the need for constant control of the disease, and assisting the person in personal care routines. Careful bathing and care of the feet and teeth may prevent damaging infections.

Many elderly diabetics have chronic ill health and find some assistance by social service and home health care groups helpful. Some who are unable to continue living in their homes, caring for themselves, consider moving into sheltered care facilities. Elderly persons living in retirement hotels, sheltered care homes, or nursing homes should make their diabetic needs known to staff nurses and others in charge so that meals and lifestyle will be conducive to control the disease.

Special Concerns of Male Diabetics

Impotence, generally defined as a man's inability to achieve and maintain an erection of the penis during sexual intercourse, is common in nondiabetic as well as diabetic men. Impotence has many causes, including emotional ones such as anxiety and fear. It can result from an organic problem, such as systemic or vascular disease or a hormone deficiency. It can happen because of neurological reasons, including brain disease or damaged nerves. Abuse of alcohol and other drugs contributes to impotency. Sometimes side effects of certain medications cause temporary impotency.

While physicians say that there is a higher frequency of impotence in males with diabetes, only some diabetic men notice impotency or become impotent as a result of their diabetes. When nerve endings are affected by the disease, however, reduced ability to achieve erection will occur. Vascular problems such as hardening of the arteries also contribute to the inability to achieve and maintain an erection, because an adequate supply of blood must flow to the penis.

Your health care team will meet with you and your partner to talk about your adjustments, both psychological and physical, to any changes in your physiological function. Some of the aspects they will probably mention are as follows:

- See your physician right away if you are experiencing impotence. It is possible that the condition is occurring as a response to some other factor and not your diabetes.
- Reduce or eliminate use of alcohol. This may alleviate the impotence.

- Sometimes impotence results as a side effect of medications. What medications are you taking? Perhaps they can be substituted for others with fewer side effects.
- What emotional factors are involved in your current situation? How was your sexual relationship before you had diabetes?
- If decreased pelvic blood flow is responsible for preventing blood flow to your penis, vascular surgery might be recommended, and for some a prosthesis might be recommended after thorough evaluation and family counseling.
- More attention paid to diet, well-balanced meals, and weight control may assist in a return of potency. Ask your physician and health care team to reevaluate your meal plan and other lifestyle factors that may affect your potency. Many men have found the condition reversible, and if you have it, you may find it reversible, too.

Emotional Factors and Diabetes

Coping with diabetes will be an ongoing challenge for you as well as for members of your family. Many feelings will enter into acceptance of the diagnosis. There may be some anger, guilt, or anxieties, both expressed and unexpressed. It is important for you, the diabetic, to discuss these feelings with those who love you. If it is your child who is diabetic, it is important to encourage discussion of these factors so that the child understands that having such feelings is part of the coping procedure.

Stable mental health is important for proper control of diabetes. Emotional stresses affect secretions of hormones that may counteract or interfere with the helpful effects of insulin. However, stresses cannot always be avoided easily. It is part of the human condition to react in different ways to different situations. More stress results at some times than at others. Situations that you meet calmly at one time may plunge you into turmoil at another. Your health care team will discuss dealing with the emotional component of your treatment plan. Your emotional needs and problems will be considered along with your menu plan, exercise plan, and therapy by insulin and other medications. Health professionals have had experience in helping diabetic patients cope with emotional responses to their illnesses, and their backgrounds can help you deal with your current concerns and those of your family.

Problems such as consistently mishandling the food plan, refusing to take insulin injections, consciously overeating, and suffering from depression occur in some diabetics. Health care professionals know that these situations can be handled well with the support of parents, spouses, or significant others. As you become acquainted with your health care team and how they can help you, you will begin to feel freer to discuss details about your diabetes or the disease of someone you love. Your team will help you find ways to approach everyday problems so that solutions can be found quickly and a plan of compliance with physicians' instructions can be followed more easily. When the person with diabetes appreciates the short- and long-range goals of therapy compliance seems easier and becomes a part of everyday life.

Your health care team will have many constructive ideas for you and your family. For example, they may encourage participation in a family therapy session to learn about family coping mechanisms along with other families with diabetes. Such groups foster exchanges of helpful ideas concerning the practical aspects of diabetes. They may suggest that you use the "buddy system," working with another diabetic to reinforce support and provide a model for adjustment to life with diabetes. Finally, your health care team will identify existing support systems. They will probably tell you about groups run by your local American Diabetes Association or Juvenile Diabetes affiliate, hospital, or community health department and the availability of social workers trained in diabetes counseling. Being aware of existing services is the first step toward obtaining assistance.

Hugs Help

Your needs for love and emotional support are the same as those of nondiabetics. Your health care team will help you balance these needs with the special features of your diabetic lifestyle. A combination of acceptance, understanding, and teamwork will help you and those you care about live a happy life.

10

The Price You Pay

Diabetes can be a costly disease. But it doesn't have to be. The purse strings are in your hands. You can control the costs of diabetes with your own preventive care and by following your physician's recommendations for diet, exercise, good mental outlook, and, if necessary, medication.

You will be able to measure some of your costs in dollars—the costs of equipment, insulin, syringes, medication, health insurance, hospitalization, nursing home services, doctors, and other professional services—but you can't measure the savings you will realize by preventing complications and controlling your disease. By preventing prolonged illness and premature death, you can save yourself and those you love countless hours of physical discomfort, uncertainty, anxiety, and anguish.

If you have diabetes, you will want to guard your health carefully because your chances of having other health-related problems are greater than those of nondiabetics. For example, some health experts say that about 8 out of 10 of all diabetics may have at least one other additional chronic condition, and 6 out of 10 can have three or more chronic conditions. About 2 out of 10 can have three or more chronic conditions. About 2 out of 10 have some form of heart disease and/or high blood pressure, about 4 out of 10 have kidney problems, and about 1 out of 10 has serious visual disability. These data are, however, a result of years of less aggressive care of diabetes. It is anticipated that these figures will be reduced sharply as tighter diabetic control is achieved through the improved methods and goals for diabetic management.

Hospital costs are higher for diabetics, too. According to the World Health Organization diabetics with complications tend to remain in the hospital three days longer per hospital stay than diabetics without complications. Among elderly diabetics 14 percent have been bedridden for an average of six weeks each year.

Save Your Health and Your Job

The costs of diabetes affect the economy of our nation as well as you and your family. There are at least 11 million people with diabetes in the United States (about 5 percent of the population). Estimates show that diabetes costs the nation more than $6 billion each year as a result of loss of productivity due to disease and death and direct costs reflecting expenditures for medical and related services. You can protect your own future earning capacity and your contribution to the productivity of the nation by protecting your health and saving your job *now*.

Statisticians estimate than more than 32,000 work years are lost by employed persons with diabetes because of disabilities related to their disease. That adds up to more than $400 million each year.

Diabetes isn't expensive just for employed people. Persons who stay in the home account for a great deal of productive activity in this country. Many are disabled by the complications of diabetes and cannot perform these essential functions. It is estimated that at least 21,000 work years and $65 million are lost in the households of America each year because of diabetes.

Begin Your Savings Program Now: Guard Against Hypertension

You can achieve short- and long-term savings by starting right now. You can take the first step in your personal campaign to avoid serious, unmeasurable costs by understanding them. Knowing what you are saving will encourage you to take the next step and plan each day to include a proper balance of diet and exercise. Current evidence strongly suggests that complications of diabetes—threats to life—can be prevented or greatly reduced by general good health measures.

One of the most important aspects of your new savings program will be to guard against hypertension (high blood pressure). This is important because hypertension and diabetes have several things in common. First, hypertension occurs more frequently in obese people; so does diabetes. In fact, in non-insulin-dependent diabetes those extra pounds may be a factor in the development of hypertension. A reduction of weight can mean control of your diabetes as well as your hypertension. Also, hypertension is more common in older people, and so is diabetes. For reasons not entirely certain both diseases affect more people in later life than during earlier years, but both diseases can be controlled in many cases through changes in lifestyle at any age.

Although hypertension is more common among diabetics than among nondiabetics, having diabetes does not mean that you will have high blood pressure. Nearly 35 million people in the United States with or without diabetes have hypertension. But, because hypertension can have so many effects on your vital organs, it is important to have it checked frequently so that you can do something about it if it becomes even mildly elevated. Usually you can't tell whether your blood pressure is high unless it is checked with a blood pressure measuring device. Generally high blood pressure offers no warning signals and gradually damages your vital organs.

In some cases diabetes, high blood pressure, and kidney disease are linked closely. Experts don't always agree on the sequence in which these problems occur. High blood pressure can cause the walls of the blood vessels in the kidney to change and block some of the flow of blood, resulting in damaged kidney tissue. Also, diabetics who have kidney disease often develop high blood pressure as a result of the impaired function of their kidneys. Because the problems of diabetes, hypertension, and kidney disease are so closely interrelated, preventing or controlling one helps reduce the complications of others.

Why is Hypertension Dangerous?

Hypertension does its damage by hastening the development of atherosclerosis. When this happens fatty deposits harden in the walls of the arteries and prevent blood from flowing smoothly throughout your body just as a clogged garden hose prevents a smooth flow of water from reaching your lawn.

Why treat hypertension? Studies have shown that hypertension may shorten life by 20–30 years. Experts say that half of all heart attacks and two-thirds of strokes occur in people who have high blood pressure. Appropriate treatment can result in fewer and milder effects.

When high blood pressure leads to hardening and blockage of arteries in the heart, heart attacks or severe pain can result. With hardening of the arteries the heart may not be able to continue to pump adequately and the lungs and other body tissues may become congested. When the body retains fluids a person may feel out of breath and tired after engaging in mild activity. When the arteries leading to the brain are clogged stroke or brain damage can occur.

High blood pressure can lead to hardening of the arteries in the legs and to poor blood circulation. When poor circulation is combined with diabetes, infection and sores on the feet and legs can be more difficult to treat and heal.

If You Do Have High Blood Pressure

If you have high blood pressure, it will be important to control it along with your diabetes to safeguard your vital organs, especially your kidneys, heart, brain, and eyes. It is important for nondiabetics to treat hypertension, too, but it's even more important for diabetics because of the combined menace the diseases present.

Your health care team will explain the significance of weight loss, if you are a little heavy, salt and cholesterol limitation in your diet, and exercise for cardiovascular fitness in fighting high blood pressure along with diabetes. If you smoke, you will be advised to stop. If these methods do not bring your high blood pressure under control, you will be advised to follow a program of drug therapy under your physician's careful supervision.

Diabetes and Hypertension Medication

If you have diabetes *and* hypertension, your physician will explain the interaction of antihypertensive medications and blood glucose levels. Because of this interaction, if you need medication, your medication and diet may be a little different from those prescribed for others with high blood pressure who do not have diabetes. Diuretics are the most widely prescribed category of antihypertensive drugs. Unfortunately, in addition to reducing your blood pressure, some diuretics may also reduce your potassium stores. Some authorities say that inadequate potassium may interfere even more with your ability to make adequate insulin. If you are advised to take a diuretic, you may also be advised to eat a diet rich in potassium (bananas, citrus fruits) or take a potassium supplement.

Some diuretics also tend to increase levels of cholesterol and triglycerides, and you may be advised to offset these effects by following a diet that includes less animal fat and fewer dairy products.

Many persons with hypertension take one of a category of drugs known as beta blockers, which influence one part of the sympathetic nervous system. They work by blocking the effects of the stimulation coming to the heart and blood vessels through a special group of sympathetic nerve fibers called beta adrenergic. These drugs decrease cardiac output by acting on nerve receptor sites in the heart. In this way they decrease the amount of sympathetic nervous output into the heart. The heart rate slows, the heart does not work as hard, less blood is pumped, and blood pressure goes down. However, the beta blockers also suppress the effect of hormones, including adrenaline, responsible for constricting blood vessels and maintaining salt and water levels in the body. Because adrenaline is also the body's mechanism for signaling development of hypoglycemia, these drugs must be used cautiously if you have insulin-dependent diabetes.

Dividends of Good Control

If you have diabetes and begin a course of medication for hypertension, your physician will monitor you closely. You will be watched to be sure that your blood sugar is under control and to determine whether you are reacting in any unfavorable way to the antihypertensive medication. If you did not monitor your glucose level at home, you may be advised to do so after hypertension is detected, and especially if you start taking an antihypertensive medication. Your medication for high blood pressure as well as other medications may cause you to need insulin if you did not need it before. If you have insulin-dependent diabetes, you may be advised to augment your insulin dose. Your health care team will explain adjustments in your routine if they are necessary.

While a comprehensive approach will be used by your health care team in controlling both diseases, what you do for yourself will be even more important than what they can do for you. You are in charge of your everyday eating habits, exercise routine, and mental attitude. Keeping these in balance will help you keep your disease under control.

Other Threats To Your Savings Plan

Hardening of the arteries in the lower extremities of the body, known as *peripheral vascular disease*, sometimes occurs in persons with diabetes. Impairment of circulation, particularly in the legs and feet, prevents infections and sores from healing. Because this condition exists in some people with diabetes, your health care team will continuously emphasize the importance of good hygiene habits, particularly care of your feet.

Leg pain, muscle weakness, and difficulty in emptying your bladder can be caused by diabetes because diabetes can affect the nerve pathways in the extremities of the body. These problems, together with others, are known collectively as *neuropathy*, or diseased nerves. Some authorities say that more than 200,000 persons with diabetes in the United States have some symptoms of diabetic neuropathy. Again, careful control of glucose levels can prevent or reduce the severity of these complications.

In the retina of the eye diabetes can damage vision by causing the blood vessel walls to thicken, become obstructed, rupture, and bleed onto the surface of the retina. The lack of blood in the tiny vessels in the eye and the spilled blood cause scarring and lead to damaged vision. According to the American Diabetes Association diabetes is the leading cause of new cases of blindness in adults over age 45 and is 25 times more common in people with diabetes than in the nondiabetic population. This complication can be avoided through careful control of diabetes as well as hypertension. Subtle changes in your eyes, if they occur, can be detected by your physician. That is one of the many reasons for frequent checkups by your health care team.

Planning Your Budget

Some costs related to care of your diabetes can be calculated so that you can figure them into your day-to-day expenses. You may want to consider ways to save on your special equipment, insulin (if you have insulin-dependent diabetes), doctor bills, and food costs.

Equipment

What equipment for self-care will you need? How much will it cost? Prices will vary depending on your sources of supply (retail drugstore, wholesale health care supply company, or hospital-based pharmacy) and the quantity you purchase. Your health care team will be able to advise you on sources of equipment that can be purchased at a savings.

Equipment for Self-Care for Non-Insulin-Dependent Diabetics

- Urine- and blood-testing materials for glucose and ketone bodies

- Book and pencil or chart for recording results of tests and your body weight
- Oral hypoglycemic agents (if prescribed by your physician)
- Candy or other quick sources of carbohydrates

Equipment for Self-Care for Insulin- Dependent Diabeties

- Urine- and blood-testing materials for glucose and ketone bodies
- Book and pencil or chart for recording results of tests and your body weight
- Insulin as prescribed (as well as a cool place for storage)
- Syringe and needles; carrying case
- Cleansing agent and sterile cotton
- Candy or other quick sources of carbohydrates
- Glucagon ampules for injection
- Identification tag (bracelet, necklace, etc.)

Insulin

How much does insulin cost? This varies, depending on the manufacturer and the preparation ordered for you. In general, however, purified pork insulin is more expensive than mixed beef and pork insulin. Pure beef insulin may be even less expensive; in some pharmacies you might be able to save a dollar or more per bottle by using all beef insulin instead of the usual beef and pork insulin. Beef insulin, unfortunately, is less like human insulin than pork and may alter your diabetic management. Its use should be reviewed with your health care team.

Is it as effective to use the less expensive insulin? Perhaps. Your physician will advise you about which type of insulin to use. Some people may use the beef insulin, and others are better with pure pork insulin alone. Because changing from one type of insulin to another may cause a significant change in your blood sugar control, however, you might have to increase or decrease your dosage. One insulin may act for a longer or shorter time in your body, and even your physician cannot predict exactly what will happen. That is why close monitoring by you at home and by your physician in the office will be necessary if you do change insulins for any reason.

If you do change, you will probably want to monitor your

glucose level at home even more closely than you did before. Plan to make the changes at a time when such close monitoring will be convenient. For example, it would be best not to change just before going on a vacation, starting a new job, or beginning school or at any other time when a change in control would be particularly inconvenient or when close monitoring may be inconvenient.

Will the bioengineered insulin that is chemically identical to human insulin be less expensive? The answer isn't really clear yet. It depends largely on the quantities that will be produced and the demand for it. However, changing to human insulin may cause the same problems that switching between beef and pork insulin now cause. Physicians say it is too early to recognize any significant advantages in using human insulin.

Doctor Bills

How often will you have to visit your physician's office? With rising costs of health care visits to physicians' offices can be a major expense, especially if you have to pay out of your pocket each time you go. You will want to have regular checkups to be sure your diabetes is under control. How often will depend as much on what you do for yourself as on what your health care team advises. If your diabetes is under good control, you will not have to visit your physician as often as when it is not under control. And, of course, keeping your disease under control will reduce the need for hospitalization. It will be much less costly to be checked routinely at your physician's office than to risk the need for hospitalization, lost time from work, absence from family, uncertainty, and anxiety.

Health Insurance

Does your health insurance cover the expense of repeated hospitalization for complications of diabetes? Does your policy cover outpatient visits to your physician's office for checkups? Does it cover expenses of repeated blood sugar and other tests?

Some policies do cover self-tests under major medical coverage.* Others do not. Health Maintenance Organizations (HMOs) may cover more of the costs of outpatient care and tests with fewer deductibles than more traditional reimbursement or indemnity health insurance policies do. Quality of care within your economic capabilities should determine the system you choose. These are some of the aspects you will want to look at closely while you are working to bring your disease under control to ensure your future good health.

Life Insurance

Do life insurance premiums go up for people with diabetes? Premiums usually are altered by any chronic condition or risk factor indicated on a physical exam report. In some cases there may be limitations of coverage. Because there are so many variations among individuals and insurance plans, this is a question you will want to discuss with your insurance agent. Your degree of control may be questioned by your agent. Generally diabetes that is under control will be your best "life" insurance.

Food

Will your food bills go up? Will you have to buy special foods for yourself? If you are a well-informed consumer, the answer to both questions is "no." Most physicians say that diets for diabetics are not special diets; they are diets for good health. Most of the time you should eat the same foods as other members of your family. However, you will have to watch the quantity you eat as well as the caloric and sugar content (as they also should). While many manufacturers label their foods sugar-free, you have to watch labels to learn how many calories are in each serving and what other ingredients, such as salt, are contained in the products. Nutritionists who advise patients with diabetes may say that many foods, such as canned fruits, can be drained from their syrupy liquids and used carefully by persons with diabetes as well as nondiabetics, but fresh fruits and vegetables that are unprocessed and that you prepare yourself are best.

*(See also Page 151)

Tax-Deductible Items

Some of the items you use for care of your diabetes may be tax-deductible. Tax laws change frequently. Check with your tax advisor to determine which of your items may be tax-deductible.

What's the Bottom Line?

Caring for your diabetes won't involve large amounts of out-of-pocket expenses that can't be factored into your weekly or monthly budget. Most people with diabetes find that by carefully purchasing equipment, insulin, and other medications; questioning their physicians about the type of insulin used; and shopping wisely for food, they can control their expenses as well as their diabetes.

Remember that coping with the high costs of the complications of untreated or poorly treated diabetes *is* expensive. It could, in fact, cost you a great deal of money. It may also cost you your life. Your physician and health care team have not overemphasized the importance of proper care. They want to help you preserve your precious good health, something money can't buy.

11
What's in the Future?

What are the chances for finding better techniques to control your disease in the future? What are the chances of future generations having less diabetes? What is being done to find a cure?

Because of current research efforts, prospects for not only treating diabetes but also preventing it look promising. Diabetes is a complex disease involving many body systems, and it interests many researchers who study various aspects ranging from the genetic details in unborn children to improved drug therapies for those who have had diabetes for many years.

Not a New Disease

Current knowledge about diabetes and its treatment has evolved over the thousands of years since the disease has been known to man. Medical historians say the ancient Chinese diagnosed diabetes by tasting the patient's urine to determine if there was too much sugar in it. Persian and Greek medical writings describe symptoms of diabetes found today. Ancient treatments consisted only of strict diet, which helped only in milder cases. This treatment prevails today for many cases and may be the therapy plan advised for you.

Research in the past 100 years has led to better ways of treating diabetes. The first significant step in modern research came in

1869 when a German pathologist, Paul Langerhans, discovered that some cells in the pancreaś, known as beta cells, were different from the other cells and that they are responsible for production of insulin in our bodies. Then in 1921 two Canadian physicians, Sir Frederick Grant Banting and Charles Herbert Best, extracted a substance (insulin) from the pancreases of animals, injected it into dogs, and found that the insulin reduced the amount of sugar in the dogs' blood. In 1922 the first patient in the world was injected with insulin, and the glucose content in his blood dropped. Since then insulin has saved the lives of millions of diabetics and helped them lead productive, happy lives. It can do the same for you.

Research efforts have improved the purity and quality of insulin. And in the middle of this century substances were discovered that improve the production of insulin by the pancreas itself. These are useful in treating milder cases of diabetes. Changes in the conventional use of insulin delivery have been developed, and research efforts regarding the means of administering insulin are under way.

Research Efforts Focus on Causes and Care

Basic researchers are continuing to hunt for information on causes and to determine better ways of controlling diabetes. They are looking carefully at the mechanisms of insulin secretion, insulin action and resistance, and glucose balance and are investigating how insulin receptor sites are altered by drugs.

Researchers think that certain individuals have an increased risk of developing diabetes. Characteristics of suscepüibility are being studied so those at risk of developing diabetes can be identified and appropriate preventive measures can be taken. Considerable research is being focused on certain viruses, reactions of the immune system, and environmental factors as possible contributors in the development of diabetes. Vaccines are being researched and tested, and some say there is hope of developing an immunization against the viruses that produce juvenile-onset diabetes.

Also, in many parts of the world, diabetes associated with malnutrition or damage to the pancreas is a continuing research concern.

Viruses

Some experts believe that certain cases of insulin-dependent diabetes may be caused by a combination of genetic predisposition, viruses, and autoimmune response (the body attacking its own cells as foreign objects). Some are studying viruses suspected of damaging the insulin-producing cells of the pancreas. Some think that known viruses, such as those that cause mumps and measles, might also contribute to the onset of diabetes. They are reexamining these viruses and seeking data on how they might lead to diabetes. In studying the relationship between viruses and autoimmunity they tentatively believe that in most cases of insulin-dependent diabetes there *is* an important interaction between viruses and autoimmunity. However, the immune system is complex, and diabetes develops in different ways in different people so that many avenues of research will continue to be explored. Scientists are unlocking the secrets of diabetes with each new discovery, and in time their efforts may yield results that will help you with diabetes. The secret that unlocks the cure is certainly the anticipated hope of all investigational research.

Malfunctioning Cells in the Parcreas

Some researchers are looking at the sensitivity of the beta cells in the pancreas to glucose and studying how the cell is affected by the concentration of glucose in the blood. They think that certain glucose-specific receptor cells are affected by multiple factors. In those with diabetes these receptors are less sensitive or less available for insulin effect. This reduced sensitivity is an inherited factor. Scientists hope to find a way to repair or improve the gluco-receptors of insulin-utilizing cells.

Answers to questions concerning the activity of these cells may result in techniques for preventing diabetes in future generations.

The pancreas in an unborn child may be affected by elevated blood sugar in the mother. According to the World Health Organization increasing numbers of children throughout the world will have pancreatic dysfunction, and in more of these cases than previously the pancreas will be affected and diabetes may result. They say these infants can be genetically marked for diabetes. Current efforts are directed toward offsetting the effects of this progressive development of diabetes through better education, improved nutrition, and earlier management of diabetes, particularly in potentially childbearing women.

Artificial Pancreases and Pancreas Transplants

Many researchers have tried to develop a system with an artificial pancreas to maintain normal glucose levels in which administered insulin is controlled by the prevailing glucose level. They have developed units in which blood is taken continuously, and its glucose content is determined by a computerized device. Another computer then calculates the insulin requirement and, utilizing a pump, injects the appropriate amount of insulin. Such systems are expensive and appropriate only for short-term studies and currently have little value to the average person with diabetes. Based on their knowledge of such equipment, however, researchers are hoping to develop smaller, implantable systems to measure glucose and automatically administer insulin.

Scientists have found that transplantation of a healthy pancreas in animals with diabetes can lead to favorable changes in the capillaries of the diseased animals. Whole pancreas transplants in man, however, have been tried but are not common. One of the problems involved is rejection of the graft. Treatment to prevent rejection is long-term, expensive, and currently limited to experimental study. However, efforts to transplant small portions of the pancreas or islet cells are promising, and scientists are somewhat optimistic about the future of implanting pancreatic cells in persons with diabetes.

Insulin Pumps

Efforts to develop an artificial pancreas led to the development in the late 1970s of small, portable insulin pumps. Three systems are currently available in such pumps: open, closed, and a combination. Some diabetologists say the ideal would be a completely closed system that includes a glucose sensor to reflect the constant blood sugar level, which would be connected to a computer that would move insulin out of a reservoir into the circulatory system on demand. Such a unit could keep diabetes well controlled. The major difficulty in developing this system has been devising a dependable sensor. Semiclosed systems or open systems would have pumps that can be programmed or adjusted by the patient to release doses of insulin based on self-monitored glucose levels.

These devices are constantly being improved. At this time several such units are available. Advantages of these methods over self-administered multiple insulin doses are being evaluated in many research centers of the world.

Several implantable pumps have also been developed. These units utilize refillable insulin reservoirs and techniques for adjusting dosage. Generally, insulin pumps are about the size of a package of cigarettes. Their designs are constantly being modified.

Advantages of the pump are that a continuous infusion of insulin throughout the day and an extra dose at mealtime can be programmed and allows the body to use its sugar more normally at all times. The pump permits constant nighttime dosage. In some studies persons using the pumps were reported to have maintained better control over their diabetes. These developments should reduce risks of developing complications from diabetes.

Pumps usually require having a needle implanted in the wearer's skin. It must be changed or removed frequently for activities or every two to three days to avoid damage or infection. Disadvantages of the pump are that persons using it must change the needle position every day or every several days, they must be careful that the needle does not become dislodged, and they must remember to set dials appropriately before meals and at other times. Some think the pump is bulky and uncomfortable. In some studies people with diabetes did not think that the pump provided an easier means of taking insulin. However, some agreed that the pump permitted them to achieve better control. Researchers say that the pump treatment is not appropriate for most and is still a research device.

If you have insulin-dependent diabetes, you may want to ask your physician if the pump might help you maintain better control of your diabetes. Ask if your physician has been adequately trained in use of pumps so you can be instructed in use of one if it is recommended to you. Also, make certain that there is a complete 24-hour support team available to you. Diabetologists advise that only patients who have access to such 24-hour support should use pumps.

Artificial Insulin

Recently, through bioengineering techniques, human insulin has been produced and approved for use in humans. Previously commercial insulin came from beef and pork. Until this achievement many scientists were concerned that demand for insulin might someday exceed the supply. As human insulin is produced by more pharmaceutical manufacturers in larger quantities, it will become less expensive and its use will become more widespread. There are also some other advantages. Patients using the engineered insulin are now being studied to observe any extra benefits not provided by other types of insulin.

Researchers are attempting to determine whether all new diabetics or insulin-using diabetics such as those with pregnancy diabetes or drug-induced diabetes may have better results using the purer or chemically produced insulins. Until this is determined, however, you should discuss the effectiveness, cost, and availability of insulin with your doctor if you are interested in changing your type of insulin.

Pregnancy and Childbirth

Diabetes researchers are seeking better ways to prevent serious birth defects and postnatal problems that sometimes occur in infants of diabetic mothers. Research centers on helping every diabetic woman who wants to give birth to have a healthy infant.

Researchers are hoping that improved home blood-testing devices and better insulin delivery programs will become more widely used so that expectant mothers can maintain better control of their blood sugar.

Also, diabetologists hope that expectant mothers can improve their blood sugar levels before conception occurs and thus guard their unborn babies against possible serious birth defects that high blood sugar can cause during the first weeks of pregnancy. With better management and techniques for administering insulin, more diabetic mothers will be able to carry their pregnancies more normally and fewer cesarean sections will be necessary among them. Methods to monitor fetal health are improving, and pregnancies among diabetics will be subjected to decreased risk under the physician's careful supervision.

Treatment Through Diet

Goals of weight normalization and adequate diet remain of primary importance in controlling diabetes. Nutritional researchers are looking at the effects of various aspects of diet on the way diabetics utilize the foods they eat. Some researchers are questioning the advisability of low-carbohydrate diets. Others are suggesting lowering the ratio of saturated to unsaturated fatty acids. Trials of these diet plans are under way, and eventually results may help others with diabetes control their disease in better ways.

Some scientists say that a deficiency of fiber in the diet may affect insulin availability. Also, they suggest that an increased fiber content in the diet may improve blood glucose control in those who have diabetes. Some data indicate that the addition of certain components of fiber improves control of glucose and reduces the need for insulin and oral antidiabetes agents.

What's Ahead For You?

Researchers now have many tools and techniques for measuring and controlling diabetes. The development of manufactured insulin, home glucose monitoring, islet cell transplantation, and better control of diabetes, as well as the possibilities for identifying possible viruses responsible for triggering the onset of diabetes, may have long-range benefits for you. How these techniques can specifically help you can best be determined by your physician.

While long-term studies continue on these and other prospects for enabling you to control your diabetes better, the experts still emphasize that *you* are the most important factor. They say that no matter how sophisticated the technology created in the laboratory becomes, each person with diabetes will want to devote careful attention to diet and exercise. Diet and exercise with proper insulin availability and effective emotional coping will continue to be the primary ways to control diabetes.

12

Resources

In addition to your physician and health care team, there are many resources available to help you and to provide information about living with diabetes. Many organizations provide brochures, newsletters, and reading lists. Some publications are available in a Spanish edition.

Your public library and local bookstores have books to help you live better with diabetes. Educational films are available from several service organizations. Gifts appropriate for individuals with diabetes are available from many sources. Following are details on several types of resources.

Brochures, Films Membership and Subscriptions

American Diabetes Association

The American Diabetes Association provides a wide variety of information on how you can stay well and active and become an effective partner with your physician and health care team. Many educational brochures are available for a small charge. You may want to write for a complete publications list and choose the ones that interest you.

A bimonthly magazine, *Diabetes Forecast*, is available by subscription.

Additionally, the American Diabetes Association has a series of films to help individuals with diabetes better understand their disease. You can borrow the films, which range from 8 to 24 minutes in length, without charge beyond the cost of the return postage.

Also, you can inquire about your local chapter of the American Diabetes Association. There are branches or affiliates in most states. These organizations make additional information available to persons with diabetes, plan programs of interest to diabetics, and provide a link between patients and physicians treating individuals with diabetes.

Check your local telephone directory for a branch of the American Diabetes Association or contact:

American Diabetes Association
2 Park Ave.
New York, NY 10016
(212) 683-7444

Juvenile Diabetes Foundation

This organization supplies information and services for juvenile diabefics. It will also provide details on the Association of Insulin-Dependent Diabetics (AIDD) programs, which offers counseling for individuals with recently diagnosed insulin-dependent diabetes. The Juvenile Diabetes Foundation will refer you to your local chapter and provide information on support groups for parents of diabetic children within these chapters. You may write to the foundation for a list of brochures of interest to parents of diabetic children, diabetic children, and diabetic women interested in having children.

Juvenile Diabetes Foundation
23 E. 26th St.
New York, NY 10010
(212) 889-7575

National Diabetes Information Clearinghouse

The NDIC prepares a bimonthly newsletter. You may be added to its mailing list and receive the newsletter without charge. The clearinghouse also provides a free bibliography regarding diabetes.

National Diabetes Information Clearinghouse
PO NDIC
Bethesda, MD 20205

American Heart Association

A wide variety of literature on heart-related topics is available from the American Heart Association. Of particular concern to those with diabetes may be the publications regarding high blood pressure. Materials are written at various reading levels. Write and ask about materials in your specific area of interest.

American Heart Association
National Center
7320 Greenville Ave.
Dallas, TX 75231

High Blood Pressure Information Centre

Reprints of articles, informational brochures, and handbooks relating to high blood pressure are available. Many of these will interest the individual with diabetes.

High Blood Pressure Information Center
120–80 National Institutes of Health
Bethesda, MD 20205

Services for the Visually Impaired

American Foundation for the Blind

This nonprofit organization provides a wide variety of publications, aids, and services for the visually impaired. Its free publications include several of interest to individuals with diabetes. You may want to write for its catalog of publications explaining aids for diabetics, including watches, canes, kitchen aids, and devices that enable blind diabetics to measure and administer insulin.

The American Foundation for the Blind
15 W. 16th St.
New York, NY 10011

The New York Association for the Blind

This organization records *Diabetes Forecast* (a publication o the American Diabetes Association) in full. Cassette tapes are free when picked up; there is a charge for mailing. The association will record an issue of *Diabetes Forecast* for you without charge if you send a blank 90-minute tape. You may write for the association's list of books and pamphlets, available in regular ink print or Braille.

The New York Association for the Blind also provides the services of the Low-Vision Clinic, staffed by ophthalmologists and optometrists who work with insulin-dependent diabetics in demonstrating a variety of equipment available for individuals with low vision.

New York Association for the Blind
111 E. 59th St.
New York, NY 10022

Diabetic Self-Care Foundation, India

This organisation has dedicated its services to diabetic patients. It has been created and supported by the patients themselves with the sole aim of helping all those who suffer from this prolonged complicated disease. This organisation aims at patient's education programme, training in self-care, diabetes detection drive, special treatment of complications, care of underpriviledged and many other such programmes. *Diabetic News*—a quartely magazine published by the foundation is available by subscription. Please contact:

The Editor
Diabetic News
C/o Diabetic Self-Care Foundation
13, Sheik Sarai, Phase-I, Malviya Nagar
New Delhi-110 017.

Insurance for Individuals with Diabetes

'Mediclaim' policy holders are admissible for hospitalization and domiciallary hospitalization benefits by the Insurance Companies of India. This policy is available with all the Insurance Companies which are subsidiaries of General Insurance Corporation of India. They are:

1. The New India Assurance Co. Ltd.
2. The Oriental Insurance Co. Ltd.
3. National Insurance Co. Ltd.
4. United India Insurance Co. Ltd.

Please contact the local office or the agens of the company.

Gifts for Those with Diabetes

Helpful Hints

The American Diabetes Association advises against giving a person who has diabetes "dietetic" candy, cakes, cookies, and breads. So-called "dietetic" foods are not "diabetic" foods. These may not contain sugar but are sweetened with other carbohydrates that your physician may not recommend for your diet.

Membership/Subscription

If your friend or relative with diabetes is not a member of the American Diabetes Association, you may want to give a gift of membership, which will include a one-year subscription to *Diabetes Forecast* magazine. You may write to the American Diabetes Association at the address given earlier.

Self-Help Groups

Across the country there are many organizations and telephone networks that provide mutual assistance to persons with similar concerns. Many people with chronic health problems have found that the encouragement and support of others helps them cope with their concerns in a more constructive way. In some groups professionals are paid to lecture or provide instruction. In some cases minimal costs for participation are sometimes involved.

These agencies provide free referral services for individuals seeking self-help groups about particular concerns. You may be interested in groups focusing on issues other than diabetes. For example, if you want to overcome depression or meet others with visual handicaps, these referral centers can direct you accordingly.

Also, you may want to contact your local hospital, health department, or community center regarding groups of interest, such as those for persons with stress-related disorders or groups that concentrate on a variety of subjects ranging from seeking employment to meeting potential mates. As a means of self-help, you may want to join a group that has nothing to do with diabetes. Develop a hobby. Learn a new skill. Teach a skill to someone else. Become interested in something different from your daily work. By focusing attention on something exciting you may find that you feel healthier and can cope better with your diabetes.

Useful Addresses of Care & Treatment Centres in India

1.   Diabetic Clinic
     Post-graduate Institute of
     Medical Education & Research
     Chandigarh

2. Diabetic Clinic
   All India Institute of
   Medical Sciences
   New Delhi-110029

3. Diabetic Clinic
   Maulana Azad Medical
   College
   New Delhi-110002

4. Diabetic Self-Care Foundation
   13, Sheik Sarai Phase-I, Malviya Nagar
   New Delhi-110 017

5. Diabetic Clinic
   SN Medical College
   Agra U.P.

6. Diabetic Clinic
   KG Medical College
   Lucknow U.P.

7. Diabetic Association of India
   Maneckji Wadia Building
   127 Mahatma Gandhi Road
   Bombay 400 001

8. Research Society for Study of
   Diabetes in India
   Deptt of Endocrinology
   All India Institute of
   Medical Sciences
   New Delhi-110029

9. Diabetic Research Centre
   5, Main Road
   Royapuram
   Madras 600 013

10. Diabetic Clinic
    TN Medical College
    BYL Nair Hospital
    Bombay 400 008

11. Diabetic Clinic
     Jaslok Hospital
     Bombay

12. Diabetic Clinic
     Bombay Hospital
     Bombay

BOOKS ABOUT DIABETES

New books to help those with diabetes live full and active lives are added to the bookshelves of bookstores and libraries each week as writers develop different approaches to providing education about the disease. To keep up with the latest additions in this subject area, visit your local bookstore or library often. To get you started on a reading program, here are two suggestions.

Lodewick, Peter A., MD. *A Diabetic Doctor Looks at Diabetes: His and Yours*. Cambridge, MA: RMI Corporation, 1982.

American Diabetes Association, Inc. *Diabetes in the Family*. Bowie, MD: Robert J. Brady Co., a Prentice-Hall Publishing and Communications Company, 1982.

A wide selection of cookbooks is available. Visit your nearest library or bookshop or write Diabetic Self-Care Foundation, India for a listing of those published by the foundation.

Could you be a Potential Diabetic?

		Yes	No
1.	History of diabetes in the family?	☐	☐
2.	Are you over 40 years old?	☐	☐
3.	Are you over-weight?	☐	☐
4.	Do you eat more than people of your age?	☐	☐
5.	Do you feel thirsty more than other people?	☐	☐
6.	Do you pass urine more frequently?	☐	☐
7.	Do you feel run down and tired easily?	☐	☐
8.	Do you get boils or sores on your body?	☐	☐
9.	Do wounds take longer in you to heal?	☐	☐
10.	Have you changed glasses more frequently?	☐	☐
11.	Any loss of weight lately?	☐	☐
12.	Women: Were your babies over-weight at birth?	☐	☐
13.	Women: Do you have vaginal itching?	☐	☐

The more "Yes" you have, the more chances you have of having diabetes.

*Source: *You Can Prevent Heart Attack* by Dr. O.P. Jaggi, published by Orient Paperbacks.

Early Detection of Diabetes is Vital Because...

... Symptoms are only minimal.

... Chances of damage to other systems is then minimised.

... Disease is easy to control.

... It can be easily treated.

... Untreated symptoms may cause more damage and other complications.

Exercise is Essential Because...

- It is can essential part of everyone's daily life including those suffering from Diabetes.

- It promotes and ensures a good health and offers. mental relaxation.

- It helps in consuming extra calories without strain on insulin requirement.

- It smoothens blood sugar fluctuations.

- It helps in burning up sugar and thus decreasing the need for insulin.

- It helps in controlling weight. Diabetics should not be over-weight.

All Cases of Diabetes Cannot be Treated with Oral Medicines Becasue...

- Tablets are not substitute for insulin.
- Blood sugar can be brought to normal by tablets only in not-so-severe cases.
- No amount of tablets can make up for severe insulin insufficiency in the body.

Is Insulin the Real Treatment?

- Not always. Your doctor may suggest an alternative.
- It is only a replacement treatment of deficient hormone, i.e., insulin.
- It can be considered as next best way to natural recovery.

Do's and Dont's for Diabetic Patients

Do's

- Accept the diagnosis.
- Try to learn about your disease sincerely and follow the instructions given by your doctor.
- Take your prescribed diet regularly. If offered, politely but firmly decline what you must not eat.
- Your health is more important than social embarrassment.
- See your doctor regularly for check-up.

Dont's

- Do not doubt the need for proper treatment.
- Never fall prey to unscientific miraculous remedies and offer yourself as guinea-pig for experimentation by an amateur or unqualified person.
- Do not take for granted that you cannot develop any complications of the disease, since you beleive so.
- Do not take your tablets or insulin injections rather casually; even occasional slips can lead to avoidable complication.

Glossary

Acetone: One of the larger classes of chemicals called *ketones*.

Acidosis: An abnormal condition resulting from too high a level of acids in the blood (*see* ketoacidosis).

Adrenaline: An important hormone in the body; also known as *epinephrine*. It prepares the body for emergencies by raising blood pressure, making breathing easier, speeding the heart rate, and increasing blood sugar.

Adult onset diabetes: *See* maturity onset diabetes.

Albumin: A protein found in the blood.

Alcohol: Is made from carbohydrates and is digested like a fat in the body. It provides about 7 calories per gram in its pure state. Beverages such as hard liquor, beer, and wine range in alcohol content from several percent to more than 50 percent.

Amino Acids: The basic building blocks of proteins, which link together in chains of varied lengths to produce an infinite variety of proteins. Scientists know of over 20 different amino acids.

Arteriosclerosis: A general term that describes a number of diseases of blood vessels, of which atherosclerosis is the most important to the diabetic.

Artery: A blood vessel that carries blood from the heart to the other parts of the body. Vessels called *veins* return the blood to the heart.

Atherosclerosis: Characterized by hardening and thickening of the arteries due to an accumulation of fatty substances along the inside of the arterial walls. This reduces blood flow and raises blood pressure. Atherosclerosis can be a serious complication for a person with diabetes.

Asymptomatic: Without noticeable symptoms. Diabetes is an asymptomatic disease. For this reason persons with diabetes should ·not assume their condition is entirely stable simply because they feel well.

Beta Cells: Located in the pancreas and responsible for producing the body's supply of insulin.

Blood Sugar: The level of glucose in the blood. Physicians can easily obtain the level from lab tests, and diabetics can obtain an approximation through home testing.

Brittle: A term used to describe a type of diabetes that varies from good control to poor control and shows great fluctuations of sugar levels daily. Brittle diabetics find it very difficult to control their diabetes, and they show extreme reactions to changes in glucose and insulin levels in the bloodstream.

Brown sugar: A form of sucrose that contains some molasses, which is also a sugar.

Calorie: A unit used to express heat or energy obtained from food. About 3,500 calories are equivalent to one pound of body weight. Carbohydrates, fats, and proteins, (and ᾽alcohols) are all energy sources and thus provide calories. Nutrients such as vitamins ·and minerals do not provide calories, but without them the body cannot function well.

Carbohydrates: Sugars and starches that are made up of carbon, hydrogen, and oxygen. Like protein, they provide 4 calories per gram.

Cardiovascular: An adjective referring to the heart and blood vessels.

Cholesterol: A fat-like substance that is an essential component of human cells. Too much cholesterol in the blood will stick to artery walls, clog them, and lead to atherosclerosis.

Coma: A state of profound unconsciousness. In persons with diabetes, coma may result from hypoglycemia or hyperglycemia.

Confectioner's Sugar: *See* sucrose.

Corn Sugar: A form of glucose made from cornstarch, about half as sweet as sugar.

Corn Sweetener: A liquid sugar, which, like corn sugar, is derived from cornstarch.

Dehydration: A condition resulting from loss of body fluids. To avoid dehydration one must replace fluids by drinking more liquids at times of exercise, exertion, or sweating.

Dextrose: The commercial name for glucose.

Diabetes Insipidus: A disorder in which large amounts of urine are excreted. The urine is normal and sugar is not present as in diabetes mellitus. For further information on diabetes insipidus, consult another source. This book concentrates on diabetes mellitus.

Diabetes Mellitus: A condition characterized by an excess of sugar in the blood and/or urine. It develops due to the body's inability to make appropriate use of ingested food as a result of insufficient availability of insulin. The term was derived from Greek words meaning *passing through* and *sweet as honey*. In this book diabetes mellitus is referred to simply as *diabetes*.

Diabetologist: A physician who specializes in treating patients with diabetes.

Diuretics: Drugs that act to increase urine output and lower the volume of water in the body.

Dulcitol: A sugar alcohol.

Edema: The swelling of tissues due to an accumulation of excess salt and water in the body.

Enzyme: Proteins that speed up or allow a chemical reaction in the body to take place.

Fat: One of the three main food energy sources; the other two are proteins and carbohydrates. Fat provides 9 calories per gram, more than double the caloric value of carbohydrates and proteins.

Fiber: Dietary fiber is the part of vegetables and grains that is not broken down by digestive juices in the intestine, as are other food elements. Fiber in the diet is considered important because it helps hold water in the intestine, adds bulk to stools, and softens them. It also helps regulate the time it takes for food waste to move through the body.

Food exchange: Groups of foods that, in givèn portions, provide equal amounts of nutrients and calories.

Free foods: A food containing little or no calories that may be used in limitless quantities by persons with diabetes.

Fructose: A natural sugar also known as *fruit sugar* or *levulose*. Fructose is sometimes almost twice as sweet as sucrose, or table sugar.

Galactose: A type of sugar found in lactose, or milk sugar.

Gestational diabetes: Diabetes that occurs during pregnancy. Often, diabetes manifests itself during pregnancy; sometimes it disappears after the pregnancy.

Glucagon: A hormone produced by the pancreas that raises the blood sugar level by causing the breakdown of glycogen (stored glucose).

Glucose: The form of sugar that the body uses for energy. It causes a rapid rise in the blood sugar, or blood glucose level. All starches eventually break down into glucose, as do all sugars.

Glucose syrups: Syrups that contain glucose and maltose and are made by breaking down starches.

Glucose tolerance test: A test commonly done in physicians' offices as a part of a complete examination or specifically because diabetes is suspected. The test enables your physician to chart your blood's glucose level over a several-hour period. It involves taking a small specimen of blood from your arm. You usually drink a beverage containing glucose at the start of the testing period.

Glycemia: A general term meaning *sugar in the blood. Hyperglycemia* is a more specific term meaning too much sugar in the blood, while *hypoglycemia* denotes too little sugar in the blood.

Glycosuria: A term used to denote sugar in the urine. Sugar in the urine can be measured by both doctor and patient.

Glycogen: Exçess glucose stored in muscles and the liver for future use.

Gram: A metric unit of mass and weight. There are 28.35 grams in an ounce and 453.6 grams in a pound.

Granulated sugar: A form of sucrose.

Honey: A natural syrup that comes from flowers from which bees collect nectar. It contains glucose, fructose, and water. While it has been touted as a more natural alternative to sugar, it is nevertheless converted to glucose in the body.

Hormone: Chemicals that are secreted by glands in the body and then travel through the bloodstream to affect various functions of the body.

Hyperglycemia: A high level of sugar in the bloodstream.

Hypoglycemia: Lowered blood sugar.

Insulin: The hormone produced by the beta cells of the pancreas. It acts to move glucose into the body's cells. Either the diabetic does not produce enough insulin or his cells cannot use it properly.

Invert sugar: A form of sucrose.

Islets of Langerhans: Tiny cells making up a very small part of the pancreas. Their alpha cells produce glucagon, and the beta cells produce insulin.

Juvenile diabetes: *See* insulin-dependent diabetes.

Insulin-dependent diabetes: Also known as *juvenile diabetes*. Patients require injections of insulin and a strict diet in order to control the disease.

Ketoacidosis: A sign of poor diabetic control in which toxic substances known as *ketone bodies* build up in the blood and cause it to become acidic. Ketoacidosis may induce diabetic coma.

Ketones: Bodies that form when there is a lack of insulin in the body and tissues begin to break down. Acetone, a ketone, has a distinct fruity smell, which is why a diabetic's "acetone breath" may be attributed to poor control.

Ketonuria: The presence of ketones in the urine.

Lactose: A combination of two other sugars, glucose and galactose; also known as milk sugar. Makes up about 4½ percent of cow's milk.

Maltose: Made up of two glucose units linked together. It is made during the breakdown of starch.

Mannitol: A sugar alcohol that is absorbed slowly into the blood and causes less of a rise in blood sugar than either sucrose or glucose. Derived from the sugar *mannose*, mannitol also acts as a laxative in large amounts.

Maple syrup: A syrup made from the sap of maple trees; mostly sucrose.

Maturity onset diabetes: Another term for non-insulin-dependent diabetes. Most diabetics have this type of diabetes.

Meal plan: An individual plan for a person with diabetes, which takes into account the person's eating habits, among other factors, and prescribes a diet for the number and type of exchanges to be eaten at each meal. The meal plan provides a proper measure of the three energy-yielding foods—carbohydrates, proteins, and fats—so that the person receives enough nutrients and calories.

Metabolism: The process by which the body breaks down and uses chemicals in food for energy and building blocks.

Molasses: Obtained from sugar; is made up of about one-half to three-fourths sugar.

Monounsaturated fat: Fats that are unlike both polyunsaturated and saturated fats because they neither lower nor raise blood cholesterol.

Neuropathy: A general term for any disease of the nerves.

Non-insulin-dependent diabetes: Also referred to as maturity onset diabetes. This type of diabetes does not require the person to take insulin injections to control the disease.

Obesity: A condition of being considerably overweight. Usually, anyone more than 20 percent overweight is considered obese.

Oral hypoglycemic agents: Drugs that can be taken orally in the form of pills to lower blood sugar and control diabetes. These pills do not, however, contain insulin, which is a protein and would break down under the chemicals in the mouth and digestive system.

Pancreas: A gland in the abdominal area, just behind the stomach. The gland houses the alpha and beta cells in the Islets of Langerhans, which make glucagon and insulin.

Polyunsaturated fat: Fats derived from vegetable sources. These fats lower the blood cholesterol level and are considered a favorable alternative to saturated fats, which raise the blood cholesterol level.

Polyuria: The condition of excessive urination.

Protein: A chain of amino acids. Proteins are used by the body for repair and growth. The enzymes that allow the body's chemical reactions to take place and speed them up are also proteins. Proteins yield 4 calories per gram.

Retinopathy: A general term for the disease of the retina in the eye.

Saccharin: A noncaloric sweetener that is several hundred times sweeter than sugar.

Saturated fat: Fats derived from animal sources. These fats raise blood cholesterol, and physicians generally ask patients with diabetes or cardiovascular problems to avoid them.

Sorbitol: A sugar alcohol that is absorbed by the body more slowly than glucose. It usually causes less of a rise in blood sugar. In large amounts it may act as a laxative.

Starch: A long chain of sugars that does not usually taste sweet. Through digestion starches are broken down into sugars. Examples of starch are cereal, potatoes, and pastas.

Steroids: Naturally-occurring chemical compounds that influence body metabolism. Steroids used in medicine are synthetically made.

Sucrose: A natural sugar derived from sugar beets and sugar cane. *Beet sugar, brown sugar, cane sugar, invert sugar, raw sugar, turbinado sugar,* and *table sugar* are all other names for sucrose.

Sugar alcohol: Products made from sugars that are broken down and absorbed more slowly by the body. Sugar alcohols eventually become sugar. Sorbital, mannitol, and xylitol are all sugar alcohols.

Vascular: A term that refers to the blood vessels.

Vitamins: Substances which the body requires in small quantities for normal body functions. Vitamins A, D, E, and K are classified as fat-soluble vitamins; vitamins C and B are classified as water-soluble vitamins.

Xylitol: Xylitol is a sugar alcohol that can act as a laxative in large amounts.

Home Guide to Medical Emergencies

Dr. H.J. Heimlich. M.D.,

More than 250 emergency medical situations from the comparatively trivial to the most serious, are covered in this book. The emergencies are described, the symptoms listed for easier recognition of what may be wrong; wherever possible the authors guide you to treating the problem successfully, and also indicate when expert medical help is really needed and how soon. Each entry is cross-indexed for easy and quick reference.

"An alphabetic cross-referenced guide to "emergency medical situations"—"emergency" here meaning anything from the common cold or constipation to suturing a wound, food poisoning, or appendicitis. There is good advice—like what to keep in a home medical kit, how to teach children not to be afraid of blood, etc."

Kirkus Review, USA

"... lucid, comprehensive and cross-referenced medical ready-reckoner... like thermometer, (it) is recommended for every home."

Midday, Bombay

"... (It) is recommended for every household."

Indian Express

"A very good addition in any house library."

The Hindu

Health Care in
Orient Paperbacks

Available at all bookshops or by V.P.P.

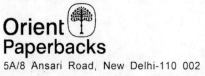

Orient
Paperbacks

5A/8 Ansari Road, New Delhi-110 002